A
ABANDONED
MIND

Charlotte Harris

To So ca,
Best wishes
Charlotte

chipmunkapublishing
the mental health publisher

Charlotte Harris

Published by
Chipmunkapublishing
PO Box 6872
Brentwood
Essex CM13 1ZT
United Kingdom

http://www.chipmunkapublishing.com

Chipmunkapublishing gratefully acknowledge the support of Arts Council England.

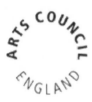

Acknowledgements

I wish to acknowledge with thanks, the help of my husband and full-time carer, Gina Smith my friend and helper and also Dr. Jonathan Bird. Also the late Dr. Harry Crow of the Burden Neurological Institute, without whom I would not have been able to write this book.

Charlotte Harris

AN ABANDONED MIND

Foreword

Dr Harry Crow, about whose work you will read a little of in this honest and compelling account, often used to refer to people with severe obsessional compulsive disorder (OCD) as being "hag ridden" by their disease. This term gives the reader some inkling of the sort of battle which Charlotte Harris has had to fight in order to emerge, so successfully, from her illness. The bravery which people who have OCD need, in order to face the world and continue to be in it, is demonstrated amply in these pages. Charlotte underwent a form of treatment, multi focal leukocoagulation, which is no longer performed. All forms of what were then called "psychosurgery " have become almost entirely unfashionable and are sometimes seen as some form of extraordinary torture carried out on people who simply have, in modern terminology, "mental health issues". This is so far from the truth as to be laughable and Charlotte's account is an important testimony to the errors of that view. Her illness was terrible and disabling and called for extraordinary measures. Charlotte's bravery and good spirit carried her through and her partnership and eventual marriage to Ian has been a vital support to her. Ian, and indeed Charlotte, have seen the psychosurgical operation as, at the time, life saving and I think in many ways it was. It allowed Charlotte enough of herself to come through and do battle with those terrible "hags" of mental illness. Ian's theory that "by the means of love and care we are reopening the good parts of the brain" seems very true; indeed with new functional imaging techniques we are starting to understand how the mind within the brain may operate and how it is affected by others about whom we care.

The reader will find this a fascinating and unusual story written with honesty and wit. It is a story of a life-long battle with OCD and of the history of the treatment of such mental illnesses over the last forty or more years. It is also a heart-warming story of human fortitude and of love which has, more or less, a happy ending.

Dr Jonathon Michael Bird
Consultant Neuropsychiatrist

AN ABANDONED MIND

Preface

Some years ago, a seed was sewn in my mind to write an account of my personal life in a detailed autobiography. Of course this meant I had to delve into my memories (which was a little difficult) due to my having undergone a selective leucotomy. I found that opening up my mind again to past experiences, exploring memories that had been buried and writing about my life exorcised a fair amount of my pent up emotions,

My life has certainly had its fair share of ups and a lot of downs. But it has surely been therapeutic to write this and I am hoping, in time to come, this record will be beneficial to a few people who have suffered as I have. Anyway, these facts are now out into the open for all to see!

I have written a record of my life, from my birth and my repressed upbringings, to my failed first marriage and finally to a happy second marriage that has reduced the affect of 'An Abandoned Mind'. All through my life people have not been able to understand what was going on in my mind (my little grey cells) and I have been subjected to 'guinea pig' treatment.

My story is one of extreme resilience and fortitude but I hope that I may be an example to others and that the fight for sanity will be never in vain!

Charlotte Harris

AN ABANDONED MIND

Introduction

This is the story of my life from the age of three and a half years when I moved from a Dr. Barnado's home, (of which I can remember nothing) to a miserable and despairing life of cruelty with Victorian foster parents. At this time (I assume because of my upbringing which was so unstable) I developed four serious mental illnesses which were not improved by my foster care and, if anything, seemed to deteriorate during my severe upbringing.

When I was eighteen years old I entered the cold outside world; this was a tough experience as I found it tough to cope with my disabilities. I sought psychiatric help and was supplied with anti-depressants, tranquilizers and sleeping tablets, all because of my continued state of anxiety.

When I was twenty three years old I got married and, of course, was still very ill. Actually, this proved to be a very bad decision as my husband did not understand me and became a fulltime alcoholic. I endured this for twenty five years and then met my second husband, a totally different man who lived with me, sympathised with my cause, supported me and has now become my full-time carer. This is Ian.

During my first marriage, I underwent brain surgery which saved my life at the time but has not diminished my illnesses and I (to this day) need constant psychiatric back-up.

I am now sixty four years of age and have somehow survived this traumatic life but only with the help and support from some people to whom I am deeply indebted.

The message is that I am still here to write this tale and you can too survive.

This is a story of my fight against the world.

Good Luck!!!   It can be done!!!!!

AN ABANDONED MIND

Chapter 1 - My Early Memories

I was born in the outskirts of Oldham on 28th May, 1943, on the kitchen floor I am told, the baby of the family, with three older brothers and three older sisters. Sadly, due to the problems in my family brought about by the war, we were split up. The youngest of the family were placed in the care of Dr. Barnardo's, in various homes in London, whilst the older members of my family went into service, as they were too old for the homes. Because of this break-up my mother was broken hearted, and eventually died of Huntington's Chorea in about 1976. My father, who was a rear gunner in a Lancaster during the war, just seemed to carry on his own life, so I never got to know him at all. In later years, when I and my sister were attending my sister's wedding, he was there with another woman and seemed very unconcerned about our welfare!

Of course my memories of the first two years of my life are very unclear, but I know we moved around and I think it was then that my life of fear began! Really I do not remember much about the war years generally, only a recurring nightmare of seeing the Matron of the home coming towards me in the dormitory, and also being locked in the toilet and not being able to unlock the door. I must admit that those memories of Dr. Barnardo's were not at all pleasant, although I do agree that Dr. Barnardo was a great man himself and that his homes provided a good way of keeping orphans off the streets at that time.

So this is how my life of fear and foreboding began!!

At that time there were many childless couples, so at the age of four years I was fostered with my nearest sister and brought to Devizes in Wiltshire. I can still remember it vividly: arriving at the garden gate with my new foster mother, still asking for my real mummy and daddy. Do you think that this was a sign of thing to come? I think so, as this seemed to be the start of what was to become what I describe as 'my years of repression'.

Anyway, here I was about four years old with my sister aged six, newly fostered (and thankfully, not adopted), leading a very austere and Victorian life. We had gas lighting, a tin bath and a toilet a few gardens away along the street. We both had to wear long woollen socks and lace-up shoes, even into secondary school. But I remember sometimes we were quite rebellious; we would take our pennies meant for the church collection (we went to high church although we were not Roman Catholic) - we would take these pennies and buy two penny chews from the shop and take a walk along the canal bank. Sometimes too, when we were given dinner money for school, we would use the money to buy sweets. And, after prayers at night, we would secrete them upstairs with us, and enjoy a 'midnight feast', but nevertheless all the time being frightened that we would be found out by our foster parents. Some prayers they were!! Still, we were only very young then and did not understand much.

AN ABANDONED MIND

I do not remember much about my primary school years, but even then I showed signs of an over-active mind and would often need to touch things repeatedly and walk away from lines in the pavement. I can now recognise this as the start of an obsessive compulsive disorder (OCD) which would come to be such a problem in my later years. I also used to have fainting fits, which I am sure were a sign of mental problems to come.

The wrath of our parents was very threatening, indeed awesome. Thank God I had my sister. We were very close, and although we were so different in personality, the blood ties were there for all to see.

So this was our life and my sister and I had to do what we were told by our foster parents. We were hit often by our mother, and quite often this was on the head. To be fair, our foster parents had had severe upbringings themselves and it was all that they had known to pass on. When my sister and I were young, we were very naive and accepted our strict upbringing because we knew that we had no choice in the matter. We accepted our insecurity and Sundays, we just used to sit on hard-backed chairs, times were very frugal and we were not allowed to sit on the sofa, this was reserved for the cat! This made us very jealous. Our foster parents seemed to idolise it (the cat I mean) and we came second in line. We used to sit on the chairs and look at the fire, and we found this very boring, although sometimes we were encouraged to read to advance our education. We had no amusements except the odd small packet of sweets as it was rationing time for some years after the war was over.

Our food regime was particularly strict. If we did not eat our dinner, then there would be no pudding; it was a sort of blackmail I suppose, but it worked!

I believe that somehow our foster parents wanted to mould us to their ways but this did not happen. They did once encourage us to be productive, attempting to try and teach us knitting. It was early days and we were not all that keen then; we ended up both tied up in a knot of wool! Well, since that time I have knitted for friends, family, sweaters, dresses, jackets and I am now attempting to knit a coat! It just goes to prove that the willingness was there, although it never surfaced for several years. Perhaps I was just a very late developer!

I slowly found my feet after a few years but it was not until later that I became a bookworm and found solace in fantasy detective novels and various historical romances. Then later I progressed to J. Arthur Conan Doyle (Sherlock Holmes) and Agatha Christie (Miss Marple and Hercule Poirot). At that time my mind was very active and open to stimulation and I was eager to improve my intellect with various reading of kinds like these. I pressed on with this informal education process, mostly to appease my parents and gain their praise.

When my sister and I erred we were hit hard (many times around the head) and we were also threatened with the poker. When we were very naughty, we were threatened with going back to the 'home', which used to put the fear of God into us. We would cry all night with this dread of going back there, so I must say we did seem to have some significantly horrific memories of those recent early years at Dr. Barnardo's.

As we were growing up, we did not like being threatened with the poker and all the other chastisements. Indeed, as my sister and I grew a little older, we started to rebel, both having friends at school who had a much easier upbringings. But it was a question of choice between the devil and the deep blue sea, a sort of 'catch 22' position.

When we left primary school we attended Southbroom Secondary Modern School and moved to a council house in Hillworth Road, Devizes where we spent the following years. Our foster parents acquired a television set at this time, but we were never allowed to touch it. We now had all the mod cons and apparently everything that we needed, except of course that which we needed most, love and happiness.

As before we were not allowed to sit on the sofa; this was still reserved for the cat!! In reality we had no forms of entertainment: no radio and we had to sit on the straight-backed chairs and were made to go to bed at about six o'clock. Later on it was extended to between seven and eight. We were never allowed to go out of the house in the evening alone, so our pleasures in life were very restricted.

We never went out except with our foster parents, but then unusually, we did find pleasure when we visited aunts and uncles. At these times our foster parents were outwardly, emotionally and pleasantly aware of us and took pride in showing us off to their relatives. So to the outside world our lives probably looked fine. We had a council house and were attending the local secondary school. We now had an inside toilet, although there was no bathroom, which meant we had to strip wash which, later on, had its problems. Our mother used to volunteer our father to assist us. He had great pleasure in doing this, touching us up and slapping our bums (in a guise to give us serious talks about life). This made us feel sick and I now feel it was tantamount to sexual abuse. After all, we were growing girls and did not really know what was going on. But there was nothing we could do about it and it carried on like that till we left. My sister and I began to dread 'wash times', so the feeling of nausea increased. In fact we later discovered that our father secretly was 'a dirty old man'.

We went to school, worked hard and led a very thrifty life. Although those first years at secondary school are a little hazy, I remember we were hit often for punishment and we were also denied all pleasures. We had set times to go to bed - and even if a film that finished at five past nine, our time to go to bed was nine o'clock, so we missed the end of the film.

I had a few close friends at school and secretly learned to ride a bike and climb trees, but was then found out and punished accordingly. One day, we could not attend school dinner and were given some money instead. All I that can remember is that we did not do what we were told and ended up at the 'tuck shop' with our school dinner money and bought ourselves some sweets and had a great time with our ill-gotten pleasures; this was one way of rebelling against our upbringing. These were early days at secondary school, and as we grew up we continued to rebel against our foster parents' ways - and things did not improve over the years!

We could not bring our friends home, as we were so ashamed of the way that we lived but later on, I used to go to a friend's house and listen and dance to 'traditional jazz' music, which was always my 'forte'. At home with our foster parents, we were not allowed boyfriends. Nor were we allowed to enhance our looks in any way at all to the extent that we were never even allowed to wear bras.

I was so envious of the freedom of my friends and spent as much time with them as I possibly could. At one time I was so aggrieved that I was not allowed to have a radio of my own that I secretly bought one and played Radio Luxembourg under my pillow at night; I prayed that I might be able to do this without the knowledge of my parents. Inevitably this led to deceitfulness and lies, which unfortunately increased as the time progressed, because we were so deprived of even the most basic things that every normal child seemed to me to have in their lives. But for me all pleasures could only take place in secret. I spent much time with a girlfriend from school, playing jazz music and dancing. I had my radio played under the pillow, whilst I prayed that my parents would not find out about my misdemeanours that were now mounting up and beginning to give me a really serious guilt complex.

While at school, we were never allowed to bring back sewing or cooking that we had achieved, therefore there were no words of encouragement from our foster parents at all as regards our interests at school. At home we could only wash up and do the dusting and polishing and we had to vacate the kitchen when cooking was in progress, so that in later years we had to start to learn to cook again from scratch.

When my sister reached puberty, I was so innocent I could not understand why my foster mother used the term 'towels' on her shopping list. It was all very secretive; my foster mother did not want me to know. But later, as always, I confided in my sister and I found out what it was all about. My foster mother did not talk to me about anything, so at that time everything that I knew about the facts of life I learned from my sister. So then, I waited for puberty to come to me, but that did not happen until I was fifteen years old. As I said before, I was a late developer. I dread to think what would have happened if I had not been prepared for puberty by my sister. I cannot imagine how I would have coped. It would have been disastrous!

As we got older we were eventually allowed out

without our foster parents, first of all only to visit girlfriends and had to be back home at set times according to the 'rules'. Then later, when we were eventually allowed boyfriends at sixteen years of age it would have to be someone our foster parents approved of although, when we invited them in, they could not sit on the sofa either.

I studied hard at school to impress my parents, but why I did this I do not know. I would be in and out of love regularly at school (usually with the teachers) and showed then that I could get very hysterical over romances. I see now this too was evidence of my emotionally instability. Indeed, I was even then showing signs of OCD, with many, many obsessive thoughts, although this was nothing to what transpired in later years.

We had many rows at home and times were hard for us. I remember once my father took his belt strap to my sister and although he did not use it and I do believe that he gained some sexual pleasure from getting her to pull her pants down in preparation. He never took a strap to me; a look from him was enough.

Whilst our fight for freedom went on, my sister and I started to go out separate ways. She left school aged fifteen to become a shop assistant. As my school results were fairly good and I wanted to become a secretary, my foster parents allowed me to go to Trowbridge College to complete the first year of a two-year course. I enjoyed this very much and left with certificates for shorthand, typing and book-keeping, skills which I progressed further when I started work in an office. Gradually I worked myself up to become a legal secretary, a challenge that makes me very proud.

Even when I was about seventeen years old and living with my parents I had a girlfriend whose house I would visit to dance and listen to jazz records. I thought a lot of her and her mother; she used to have long painted nails and I was very envious. So I grew my nails long and secretly painted them. I would then leave home for my friends' house and wore gloves to cover them up when saying goodbye to my parents. When I came back at the appointed time I would then rush upstairs, take my gloves off and dispense with my nail varnish in secret. I was growing up but still had to be deceitful in my ways but I carried on like this to have some freedom of my own. Since that time I have always worn nail varnish but, of course, no make-up until I was liberated from my parents at eighteen years old.

I later discovered that our fostering seemed to be purely mercenary, although I was allowed to attend college for an extra year when I was fifteen and achieved certificates in typing, shorthand and book-keeping. When my sister was thrown out of the house at the age of eighteen, because she had stayed out all night, my foster father cried, whether with remorse or sadness - one guess is as good as another! Anyway, he did not cry when he left me because, as I have said previously, their fostering was purely mercenary, the reason our foster parents chose not to legally adopt me and my sister, or so it seemed to me!!

My foster mother hit me on the head often and I feared her more than my foster father. When I was eighteen years of age and more mature, she hit me around the head and I hit her back!! I was angry but also very fearful, I think this may have been on of the reasons they left me although I think the financial reason was more pertinent. And when they did leave me, it was a cold parting.

Chapter 2 - Starting Work

It was when I started work that I really began to suffer rather seriously from OCD. It seemed that then there was not much knowledge about it and mine was proving to be a curious case to the doctors who tried to help me, escalating as time went on. I did not know what was happening to me with my confused, jagged thought processes, and at first I could not tell anyone what I was going through as I had no understanding myself! I feared for my sanity - my mind was like a festering ball situated inside my head! It has taken until now to decide to disclose these details to others, by writing about it like this; it shames me, and seeing it in print, it still puzzles and frightens me.

Sadly, when the problems I was having with my mind did come to the surface, I had little sympathy from my foster parents. So I threw myself into my work to try to hide my depression, but over time this really didn't help.

I had to give two thirds of my money to foster my parents, so I only had one third for my personal needs. And as the wages increased then so would my contribution to the home.

I was never allowed to wear tights as such but progressed into wearing lisle stockings when I was seventeen; my freedom was so stifled, I felt rebellion welling up inside me. I missed my sister when she left - I was so ill but had to cope with life on my own. I knew that I had to stay with my foster parents, or guardians if only for the minimal security they afforded me and of course to try to manage my fears. When I eventually had my freedom at eighteen it was like a bombshell and, where I had been so sheltered, I had to start living again by new rules. But this was freedom and I had my work and friends.

In 1960, when I was seventeen years of age, I joined the choir at St. John's Church in Devizes. I was proud of this, went to choir practice every week and sang soprano descants and 'anthems'. However, things began to fall about my feet as I would often burst into tears and could not contain my emotions. I was often overcome with emotion and found that the hymns and music would have this special effect on me. Of course, my parents never went to church and could not observe my discomfort and in some ways, I enjoyed it, with its rituals such as regularly having to starch my collars and cuffs, and it also gave me a good goal to achieve.

My parents knew I had a good voice and encouraged this but never saw the emotional turmoil I was in at this time. But then, they would not have understood as they seemed to distance themselves from it and never seemed interested enough in my plight. I was confirmed by choice at fifteen years of age and, on communion days, the choir would take the communion before the congregation. I do believe in God but sometimes wonder why he is not there for me. I have prayed often but more in mind than body. I do believe in an afterlife and think that somehow faith has carried me through the years but it has been like a tightrope walk, where the chances of falling are imminent. Nonetheless, I am so grateful for the help I have had on the way, without which I know I would not have survived. I am also indebted to my present husband who is my full-time carer and for his great love and closeness to me.

When I was going out with my Royal Air Force (RAF) boyfriends, I used to visit them at the Gliding Club at their Upavon airfield on Sundays. I was in digs then, and my girlfriend and I used to ring up in the mornings to see if there were any 'thermals'. If there were, off we would go on her scooter.

We watched the gliders take off and land and we would cook for the men and serve their meals. Anyway, sometimes they offered to take us up in a training craft. We were winched up by plane, then a hook would drop and there we were, transformed in the air on our own, with only the thermals and winds to control us, not a sound. We experienced a little 'G' force when taking a turn but I do not think that my head could have taken any more weight. Then they let us take control, with the stick up for ascending and back for descending, and from side to side to turn. Having the freedom of the elements was super, and was an experience that both of us liked to repeat. And happily It did not cost us anything. Anyhow, we went many times to Upavon and cooked for the chaps, chatted over the mealtimes, and even had time to flirt a little - those were the days!!

AN ABANDONED MIND

As I have said, when my sister was eighteen years old she was thrown out of the family home by our foster parents for staying out too long one night, and this was strictly forbidden and against their rules and regulations. My sister was packed off with her belongings and I seemed to be absolutely stunned by this situation. Then, some years later I found myself experiencing similar feelings of shock and surprise. On this occasion my foster parents said to me that they wanted to leave Devizes and return to Bath where they had lived previously, and they said I could either go with them or stay; I decided to stay with my job, and friends who I valued greatly. This leads me very much to believe that their 'fostering' was mainly mercenary. My sister Doris had gone at eighteen and the same was happening to me!!

In 1961 when I was eighteen and not long before my parents left me, I and my friends used to congregate in the 'Griddle Grill', a coffee shop where we used to discuss boyfriends, although I did not have a boyfriend at the time, my relationships with boys always having been thwarted by my foster parents. We used to sit in the coffee bar, discussing topics of all kinds with both sexes.

Having been offered a cigarette several times, I declined, naturally, then, eventually, I gave in due to peer pressure and began to enjoy smoking, but, having accepted so many cigarettes from friends, I decided it was time to buy some and pass them around. That was the beginning and I must say that I regret to say that I have smoked ever since.

Once, when I was in the coffee bar smoking a cigarette, my mother walked by. I do not know if she was shocked or just angry, but I was afraid to go home. Well, eventually I had to and I was greeted by a stony silence that lasted for a week and then I was told to try not to make a habit of it by my father, who incidentally chain-smoked and caused his own death by this action!!!

When my father died at the age of seventy five it was of arterial sclerosis plus the fact that he had a small hole in the heart. So I did not really think that he was a very good example.

I know that I regret smoking. It is a filthy habit but it was one outlet I seemed to need and of course, then it was quite acceptable. I curse the day that I started smoking and, if I had not smoked then I would be definitely financially better off by now!!

When my foster parents left me I grew apart from them and even when visiting them later on, the strict rules would still apply, even when I was twenty one years of age and over. At one time I stayed with them for a few days but, even then, on New Year's Eve they said I had to be home by twelve midnight, which I knew would spoil all the fun. Of course, I disobeyed but again was greeted by a stony silence!!

My OCD was getting worse, but I was too frightened to tell anyone of my symptoms and no-one knew what was going on in my brain. My sister had gone away and my foster parents showed little concern for me at this time and I believed that they were glad to be rid of me, as they did not seem to be able to extend their understanding to me.

So I later sought the help of a psychiatrist who assured me that I was not going mad!! It transpired that he could not be of much assistance to me, although he put me on tranquilisers and anti-depressants to try to help me. After all, this was the 1960's, and it seemed then, that little was known of this particular type of illness.

The psychiatrist put me on tranquilizers and anti-depressants and did not seem of help me very much. In 1964 at age twenty one I had the first of many nervous breakdowns. Each time I would lose a good job but somehow I would pick myself up, dust myself off and start all over again!!!!!

After a time I achieved qualifications in English lanuage, shorthand and typing, and I always seemed able to find work. Anyway, I needed the money from my jobs to exist in my own in digs and pay my expenses. I was growing up, even if a little tainted but this was how my life was going to be and I had to accept it. I really had no option. On the other hand I was isolated by my illness, while also having to learn the facts of life; neither of these options was easy for me.

At twenty years of age I was admitted to Roundway Mental Hospital in Devizes, weighing about seven stones and nine pounds; I was extremely ill with hardly any reason to live or purpose to survive.

This was one of the two breakdowns I had before I married. Each time I had a breakdown I would lose my job because of the stigma of my illness and this time, the lady who looked after me in digs, sent all my belongings back to my foster parents too.

By this time I had received further qualifications in shorthand, typing and English language and also an RSA III in typing. And I then became a legal audio typist.

When I was twenty one, after my second nervous breakdown in Roundway Mental Hospital and having been thrown out of my digs because of the terrible stigma of the illness that was instigated against me, I had to start all over again. I grew up fast, fortunately still enjoying my dancing, listening to records and having coffee in the local cafe in Devizes with all my RAF friends.

Away from my foster parents, I had to endure a severe 'learning curve', disciplining myself for not, at times staying out late. But I managed, carrying on for the next two years, going to dances, and acting normally, but feeling very frustrated inwardly. It was not easy living a double life but I took chances where I could and was quite gregarious, as this helped to hide my compulsions and inner disturbances. I had both boyfriend and girlfriends and we would sit in the coffee bar and have discussions on about everything. I certainly have no regrets about the way I lived during this period of my life.

AN ABANDONED MIND

In 1964 when I was twenty one years of age I was still a virgin. However, at that time I was going out with a Roman Catholic man. I loved him and he loved me. However, things got out of control and he raped me. I protested and put up a fight but he was stronger than I was and very much determined to succeed. After I had sex, I discovered that I was bleeding and I knew that I had lost my virginity. Anyhow, I still loved him and let him make love to me again. He was very possessive and it seemed that he wanted me to become pregnant so that I would be forced to marry him. Fortunately I did not get pregnant, due to the fact that he was a Roman Catholic it was a good thing that I did not marry him and have a family. Instead I went off to Blackpool with a girlfriend and tried to avoid him, as I no longer felt that I had any love for him. What might have been was a little frightening and it may well have been my Waterloo.

When I had lost my virginity, it was a great blow to me; I felt soiled but, as with so many things, this was a learning curve. I made a few mistakes after that with, thankfully no bad results. Then my answer became 'no' to any man after that! My first husband told me that this was his attraction to me, that I said no but, there again, that was my great mistake as explained later in my life with my first husband.

I was not in contact very much with my foster parents when they left Devizes to live in Bath but when I had one of my breakdowns and was interred in Roundway Mental Hospital they visited me. I was not really feeling up to it and I received odd reactions from both of them: my mother was cold and my father cried continually but whether this was with sadness or regret I do not know. I think that my mother could see that I had lost so much weight and that I was not the tubby girl she knew.

When I was with my first husband, we acquired a puppy 'Collie' dog. Later on when she had settled in, we took her to see my foster parents, but the dog was not allowed in the house with us and we had to leave her outside in the car. I also found this very unreasonable. After all, when they had their cat, it was allowed to rule the house, to the exclusion of us two girls. This quite obviously seemed like disapproval to me.

When I was young, my forte was traditional jazz and I co-founded my own 'Jazz Appreciation Society' of which I was secretary. I was gregarious in nature and found I could cope with my illness better this way. During this time I met and talked to several jazz bands, acquired autographs and dressed outrageously. This was my extrovert side which helped me cope with my anxiety and OCD symptoms. At this time I was seeing Dr. Waters, was taking much medication, so of course, did not drink.

This was my life now and I knew I had to hide my emotions if I was to try to have some kind of life. I courted several RAF men and in the coffee bar in Devizes enjoyed our time together, discussing anything from sex to religion.

AN ABANDONED MIND

I got to know one jazz band very well and we shared an Indian meal with each other. One musician seemed to suss out that I had problems, but it was an honour to dine with him and we parted amicably, he to his coach and me to my digs! That was most rewarding, much better than just an autograph and much more pleasurable.

I had no sexual experiences with the RAF gentlemen, they were intelligent and great company and we used to swap our boyfriends around.

The Chairman of our Jazz Appreciation Society was a homosexual. He had emotional problems too; his mother wanted a daughter so he grew up like one! He had a wonderful disposition and we stayed friends until he decided to take off and live with a boyfriend, but when I was twenty one years of age and in Roundway Mental Hospital he visited me and seemed alarmed at my situation.

Chapter 3 - Getting Married

I met Maurice Edward Somerton (or Angus as he was known to all) in 1965 in a jazz pub we both went to, as we had the same preferences in music. He appeared very debonair to me with his black beard and black hair. We met across a crowded room and later, when I refused to get in the back of his Jaguar for sex, he fell in love with me (and I with him) out of respect. Even Ian, my present husband, says that he could see why I fell for him. We were married on the 10th December, 1966.

I was married on the 10th December 1966. My husband said that it was about time we 'shacked up together', but I made him buy me an engagement ring and do the honourable thing. He had been a real Casanova during his lifetime and I was told that I would not be able to tie him down. Well, I loved him and I did tie him down, but little did I know of the sort of life I would experience with him.

Although I was not then with my foster parents, my foster father gave me away at the wedding and even now that I am in my second marriage, he preferred my first husband Angus. But even then neither knew what I was going through, so this marriage was never a good foundation for me. People would say to me 'once you are married, all will change' and later on 'once you have a baby all will change' but unfortunately none of this transpired and I am grateful to Dr. Crow for advising me not to start a family. He said that 'he would not advise it' and that was enough for me to look after myself and I thank God for him, my 'father figure'

Angus was very possessive about me, but when I was emotionally unstable he preyed on that. He also knew that I would never leave him and I did not know then what was ahead of us.

When I was first married I became pregnant but, after experiencing an enormous evacuation, was told by my friends at work that I had miscarried. I then went to a family planning clinic in Bath, while I had not told Angus about the pregnancy but, because Angus chose not to use a 'condom' I went on the birth pill which later caused me to have cervical cancer when I haemorrhaged (but this was twenty years later) and there was much to occur yet.

For the first six months of our marriage we would walk hand in hand, I would sit on Angus's lap, but we were very poor and our honeymoon soon wore off.

Although Angus had several jobs we couldn't manage, so we ended up living with my in-laws. I worked hard, sometimes having two jobs at a time, despite my breakdowns - I seemed to have some inner strength.

My father-in-law had his own business as a plumber, but, because his quotes to the County Council were too low he hardly made any money – he had too kind a heart. He was his own accountant and could be seen every night doing the book-keeping, but eventually he went bankrupt. And because of his eternal love of Woodbines, sadly at the age of seventy he died of lung cancer!

My sisters-in-law told me that I was like his fourth daughter and there was no doubt that he was a little sweet on me. While he was dying at home, I was asked to leave the room and Angus took me back to our own home until his father died then he called me back to kiss him when the final second arrived. He had been very heavily drugged with morphine and it was just a matter of time before he faded. But what I could not understand was why, if he considered me to be his fourth daughter, I had been asked to leave at the moment of his demise!! After my father-in-law died, Angus expected to inherit his father's house, but this did not happen and his eldest sister Val took over as the head of the family. The anxiety which this caused in me exacerbated my illnesses.

My father-in-law had spent all the war years as a sergeant in Africa. When he came back from the war, that was when they conceived Christine (the apple of their eye), but he was then a changed man and held a lot of bitterness inside him.

My husband had two other sisters then who I managed to get on quite well with but, as I had no children by my own choice, they could not understand my demeanour and the relationships were always a little icy.

AN ABANDONED MIND

Anyhow, when my father-in-law came back after the war years they had Christine and utterly spoiled her, I think that maybe this was a mistake in hindsight as this young daughter seemed to bring them a lot of heartache in later years. The way it seemed to me, because she was spoiled, this put the nose of the other members of the family out of joint and I must say that I sympathised with them wholeheartedly! The family showered her with everything that she could desire, and my husband did not seem to be considered to be the 'heir' any more. Later on, as I had no children, the Family Bible was given to her son instead of Angus, but he had his father's medals, which was like a token prize. But then Angus was not all that worried about his father, he just wanted to inherit the house, but ultimately, their dying father left it to Christine.

Before Christine was eighteen years of age, and instead of her getting a proper job like the majority of young women do, she fell in love with a student of Arab descent at the college that she was attending for further education. Of course, her parents encouraged this and doted on both of them, encouraging their close relationship. Later on they got married with all the approval of the family. Mind, you I was very scathing about having an Arab in the family and there were serious doubts about how and where he managed to obtain his money. It was, and always will be a complete mystery. They had a daughter who did not achieve much in life and at one time ended up on drugs. It was a fact that Abdullah was blamed for not spending enough time and love on her, but I am afraid I was out of it and not really interested.

Christine had a second child whom they called Natasha, who was born in Jordan although it seems that as she was conceived in Wales. After her birth Christine and Abdullah arrived back from Jordan and it was apparent that the baby was not well in a serious way. Soon it was discovered that they had to bring her to this county to drain her 'water on the brain'. This is a spinal condition and it was deduced that she would never walk again. Naturally, all the family was devastated at this outcome and my in-laws spent all their time loving the little girl. She always came first, at this time it was my nose that was put out of joint!!! Of course, my illness would always be a secret to all concerned but I felt that it was I who needed love and understanding.

Anyway, Natasha was a lovely little girl but to this day, she is still confined to a wheelchair and unable to walk unsupported. While she was young she made many trips to Great Ormond Street Hospital, for several treatments, but sadly there will be no cure. I strongly believe that if she had been born in this country and they had drained her brain earlier, there might have been some progress but who knows.

Well, life went on with the in-laws who treated Natasha as their own and they became quite obsessive about her, almost to the extreme. She was the daughter of their daughter and that was it.

AN ABANDONED MIND

At this time, Angus had introduced my father-in-law to drink and gambling but he seemed not to be good at either. He could not hold his drink and also lost vast amounts of money (always saying that he had made a bomb!) and he would treat the family to goodies which he could ill afford.

While we were living together at 'The Grove' Angus and I would go along to the 'Crown', the local public house which became my father-in-law's and Angus's favourite haunt. At one time I had upset Angus and he, thinking I was hysterical, struck me (that was the only time). I made out that he had knocked me out and I heard him talking in a martyr like voice about what he thought he knew of my illness. He did not attempt to pick me up and I had to gather myself together and eat humble pie. That was certainly a learning curve that I did not relish but I supposed that I had asked for that. I had wanted to draw attention to myself somehow but this had failed miserably again. I think that my feeling at that time was a mixture of jealousy and envy.

When Angus and I had our house at 9 Victoria Buildings I worked hard as a temporary legal secretary in Bristol (at one of my good times) and things were not too bad, but the nearest call for my husband, whether we were on our own or with the family, would be the nearest pub (in fact, it would be a right royal pub crawl, as I saw it!) I could not drink and it upset him greatly to buy me a coffee. In fact, I think I almost instigated 'coffees' in pubs and it now seems to have become very popular even to this day.

In 1961, when I was free from my foster parents, I began what I know call my rebellious, retro years.
I joined the current 'Traditional Jazz boom'. I became gregarious in order to cope with my illnesses and began to smoke a pipe!! I must say was very outlandish, but, as I was mainly on my own coping with this, it seemed a great thing to do at the time.

I elected myself 'secretary' and a friend of mine became the chairman and we would hire a minibus to various 'gigs' and saw and enjoyed many famous jazz bands, this was a real 'club' and we administered it as effectively as we could.

We became quite well known in many clubs. We would dress up quite ridiculously and, when dancing, whether a stomp, jive or quickstep we earned quite a reputation for ourselves at these times. At the time, I went out with quite a few RAF gentlemen and their forte was also traditional jazz. I collected autographs from all the bands I saw and also made a secretarial note of all our transactions. At the front of this book I wrote a poem:

> *Whatever your taste, enjoy the beat*
> *Modern or trad, just move your feet.*
> *Don't be afraid to let yourself go*
> *As you are all welcome where we go.*

I also used to write of accounts of good jazz sessions that we would enjoy such as:

AN ABANDONED MIND

June, 6th 1961.

The Regency Ballroom, Bath.

Contents: Acker Bilk and his Paramount Jazz Band. Playing, A Taste of Honey, Creole JAZZ, Go tell it on a mountain. Stars and Stripes (as regular) Jump in the Line and That's my Home.

Here is an extract from my notes that I wrote at the time:

'We were taken down to Bath by Mike, to see Acker Bilk and his Band which was the opening of the 'Bath Jazz Festival' at Bath.

I met Martin, Sue, (my close friend) and I dances as soon as Alex Welsh played, but not on my own for long, we were split up! From that time we were never without partners. Martin caused an exiting stir. (as usual) wearing his 'Rev' outfit turning his collar around so that he looked like a vicar. Acker said that he thought it was great and we later met his band, had autographs signed and indulged in general chit-chat with Acker and the Band.

That was just one outing, there were many more to come and I would like to say that these memories are and always will be, very dear to my heart.'

Chapter 4 - My Selective Leucotomy Surgery

Between the ages sixteen to twenty-seven, I had two nervous breakdowns, with violent mood swings called manic depression and severe anxiety. I was told the second time I went into Roundway Mental Hospital at twenty one years of age that there was nothing further they could do for me except a straight lobotomy which would leave me like a vegetable. I did not think this was very desirable at the time, so left I Roundway Mental Hospital saying that I would fight it on my own! However I was told that there may be something that could be done later, as science progressed. So, at this time I was left in a sort of void, having to suffer my illnesses with hardly any support at all except drugs which were obviously necessary for my welfare.

When I was about twenty-seven years old I was contacted by Dr. Harry Crow, of the Burden Neurological Institute in Bristol, offering me an appointment to see him with regard to undertaking of a selective leucotomy. He said that would do me no permanent damage, could improve my quality of life considerably; in fact, he suggested it had a 50-50 chance of success. However, I also learned that in this position I would be used like a 'guinea pig' for experimental purposes.

For a while I dithered about, and was advised by family, friends and foster parents not to undertake this surgery. Once I got as far as deciding I would accept Dr Crow's help and entered the Burden Neurological Institute for surgery, but I then got cold feet and returned home. After that I was extremely depressed and became so seriously ill that after three weeks of crying, I begged the hospital to admit me but they held off at first to see if I was going to rethink the matter again! They had to be sure!

I was then summoned to see Dr. Crow, who repeated that if I had the surgery he was proposing, I had a 50-50 chance of improvement. I was so desperate that I accepted against all the advice of my peers and continued to 'sign on the dotted line'. This was my decision entirely and now in hindsight, it was one of the best things that I ever did!

Dr Crow explained the process to me. He said the nurses would shave my head, insert fifty six wires into my frontal lobes with a connection on the other end of the group wires. I had the surgery at Frenchay Hospital in Bristol and was returned back to the Burden Neurological Institute the next day, with a headache that lasted six weeks. Before I had the surgery I was taken off all my medication and was kept there as an inpatient as I had severe withdrawal symptoms and was quite unwell. This was when I was introduced to Paracetamol tablets for the headache which I realised that would be compatible with my medication and I have used them ever since.

During my consultations with Dr Crow before the surgery he explained to me in some detail how my conditions seemed to come about. He suggested my illness was caused by a deep sense of insecurity that I experienced during for the first four years of my life. I couldn't disagree! Enough said!!

Dr Crow did not ask to see my foster parents at all while I was an inpatient in the Burden Neurological Institute. He just concentrated on my 'little grey cells', which seemed to be his one and only interest as regards my treatment. He was good to me and I came to look on him as a father figure. He seemed to understand what I was going through and it was a very comforting for me. Nobody else did!!!!! I had thought I was going mad with my OCD, but it was not just a normal OCD, it was obsessive thoughts (not washing hand or acute cleanliness) but it is in my mind and very hard to cope with, with mood swings anxiety and depression and also phobias.

I underwent the surgery and had to wait several weeks for the treatment (in which I had to lie down while the box in my head was plugged in and an electric current was apparently discharged through my brain. The treatment was to burn away a minute part of nerves in my frontal lobes, which I gather are the emotional parts of the brain.

Before I had surgery, I had had about sixteen treatments of convulsive therapy (ECT) at Roundway Mental Hospital and Weston Lodge Psychiatric Unit in Bath, but all that seemed to do to me was make me more depressed. I would come round from the anaesthetic (with literally the bit between my teeth) and I would be crying and exceedingly upset at this predicament and very shaken. Dr Crow said that I had not really ever responded to this treatment although I recall several of my fellow patients had responded to this treatment successfully and were apparently cured. I must have been a difficult patient!!!

I also had several 'brain readings' before the surgery. They would put several electrodes on my scalp and show me a succession of lights, some flashing; this was to test the state of my brain. I had several of these before surgery and then one while I still had the wires in, I presume to test that my treatment was complete! (I must have come out with an odd comment while I was in the hospital, and this seemed to convey to all that it was about time that my wires were removed). I do not know how this worked out but I was the patient and I so badly wanted to get rid of this interminable mental torture, because to me that is definitely what it was!!! I have since realised that this is a cross that I have to bear but all the treatment I had was very welcome in order to improve my 'quality of life' as Dr Crow put it.

While I was having treatments, as with the other 'wire patients', I was not allowed to be consulted by Dr Crow, but he was still very much in charge of me. All the doctors would attend my bedside every Monday morning to have a chat and discuss my progress. I used to cry a lot but since I have had the surgery I find it difficult to do this and over recent years my emotions have turned to anger, which I find difficult to control. It is an emotional roller coaster.......

When I had my second breakdown and at several times since, I have lost my job due to my illness; this also happened since my operation. I lost many jobs because no-one could comprehend my illness and understand what I was going through, so although I had achieved qualifications I could not maintain a good position, I could get a job but could not maintain it. Even when I married for the first time in 1966, my husband, family and friends could not understand or comprehend my suffering.

Because of my illness I could not make the commitment and, in later years, have been unable to trust anyone – I could not explain my illness as it was too complicated. This left my confidence damaged. I was classed as emotionally unstable but despite this I fought on with marriage and determined that my illness would not get the better of me. All this time (except for my then husband who could not really comprehend) no one knew what was wrong with me. I took a lot of knocks but came out fighting. After all I was a skilled person with a right to life. I was, and still am, very sensitive about my illness and very conscious of what impressions I make. I seem to be two people, one mad and one sane and I cannot find the happy medium. I find people very difficult to get on with and to talk to – I still walk around covered by an armour of confidence to protect myself, a sort of self denial. My illness was always a well-kept secret, as I knew that if I divulged it I would be ridiculed!!

I think at this point, it is pertinent to mention again

that my birth mother, although I never met her, died of Huntingdon's Chorea and one of my sisters has recently died of this illness which seems to prove a genetic disorder of my family. Does it, I wonder?

Anyhow, with great fear that this disorder would befall me as if I did not have enough on my plate, I went at the age of sixty to the Royal United Hospital in Bath to have a blood test to see if I had inherited this genetic disorder. I found that I was clear, to my great relief and continued to struggle on with my own problems.

Well – back to the surgery. When my head was shaved before the surgery, I would not look in the mirror at myself – bald – but this was a small vanity I could bypass, considering how desperate I was for this operation. Now, that I had the 'wires' in my brain I was bandaged and had to wear a headscarf. There were quite a few headscarves about, walking around in the Burden Neurological Institute. Not only did they give this treatment for neurosis, but also for phobias and various other disorders.

Although we did not much discuss our ailments, the patients got on reasonably well with each other, after all, we were all in the same boat, and it was sink or swim. Some of the other patients' illnesses were obvious but other would not talk. We all waited desperately for the call from a doctor to see us as we all needed attention to placate our personal worries.

The thought of brain surgery was terrifying – but it

was that or nothing. My husband didn't understand, nor did my in-laws. There weren't unsympathetic by choice, they were just ignorant.

The Burden Neurological Institute was an extremely pleasant hospital and was treating people with severe mental illnesses. A day's routine would include a cup of tea in bed followed by an exodus to the breakfast room. We would partake of breakfast, receive our personal drugs, which we only took if we had eaten our breakfast – and then we would go back to the main building!

Then, for those who wanted to, they would go to our day room, smoke cigarettes and talk freely with each other, as some would be summoned to see their prospective consultants, or nurses for a dressing to be replaced, and so on, if required.

Some patients would attend occupational therapy, which most found very comforting and rewarding and then we would - which was also described as 'occupational therapy' - obtain the keys to our personal responsibility (the canteen) open it up, stock with supplies and serve drinks to all and sundry.

Among the range of patients at the Burden Neurological Institute there would also be a few patients suffering from epilepsy. They would quite often have 'fits' which we soon acclimatised ourselves to and the staff were always there to allay any discomfort which we might suffer because of these.

AN ABANDONED MIND

If any of us were going home for a short spell then we would be titivating ourselves up and having baths and getting ready for this motion. This of course would be a positive omen!

This all contributed to a pleasant and appreciative in patients experience and left us all with an abiding memo of being a patient at the Burden Neurological Institute.

Some days would be 'out-patients day' for the consultants, as well as seeing us as this was a very busy hospital and we would often have to walk through the waiting room where the outpatients were waiting, some of us with our headscarves on, to our various wards and buildings of occupation.

I am afraid that quite a large amount of my memories in the Burden Neurological Institute seemed to have been lost in transit but these are a few of the memories that will abide with me for the rest of my life, and I am sure that this is similar to hundreds of patients who were treated as inpatients there!

Well, I had taken my paracetamol for about five weeks for my severe post operative condition, I was ready for my treatment and for my twice a week plug-in. There was always a doctor present with me at this time and while undergoing treatment, I felt an odd 'floating sensation' but, of course, I really did not know what was going on!!

After I had treatment, about twice a week, then I

had to be confined to my bed to rest for about an hour and was not allowed to walk around the wards until the staff drew my curtains open and allowed me to integrate with the other patients in the ward.

As I have said, one of my treatments at the Burden Neurological Institute was occupational therapy and this was where I learned to become a good seamstress. I wore one of the dresses I had made when I was discharged, some seven months later – with a full head of hair!!

The staff in the Burden Neurological Institute were wonderful. There were not many of us and we all needed individual help and advice from them. One of the rules at mealtimes was 'if you do not eat your meals then you had no medication so we were not allowed any loss of appetite no matter how you felt and, of course, the food was very good. We also were told repeatedly by the sister with all our cases that all our cases were a question of 'two steps forward, one step back' and this was very comforting to us in our state of need. Despite this, we were told that progress would be slow but positive. We all had our crosses to bear, but everyone's illness was a secret of their own and we just got on with it, I think that this would be classed as a matter of 'medical respect'.

The Burden Neurological Institute was also treating phobias, which I also have later developed, epilepsy and other disorders. The epileptics were treated with drugs, but still there were disturbed days and nights. But, of course, this was not my business but I tried to help with the other patients to the best of my ability.

Next to the Burden Neurological Institute, there was Stoke Park Mental Hospital where patients were quite seriously ill. And the noises that emanated from that place were sometimes quite alarming. But off course these people were compulsorily institutionalised and were pretty serious cases. One of our voluntary occupational therapy activities was to open the local 'canteen' so that we could have drinks, eats and a talk if so desired. Some of the patients who came to the canteen were from Stoke Park Mental Hospital and by their mannerisms frightened us to death. We were all so gullible but of course ours was a nervous illness and we hoped that that set us apart and none of us would really allow ourselves to be this depressed!

After I had had several treatments I seemed to be making no progress (or so I thought) and I became very depressed. I wanted to get better so badly that I took an overdose of Neulactil tablets but this was really a cry for help and I told the staff about what I had done. I did not really want to die and I was then supplied with several glasses of salt water which made me very sick, of course, in order to bring up the tablets. Because of the strength of these tablets I was then rather relaxed and slept greatly – it was a wonderful feeling but of course, I would not be able to live like this permanently. I was sick for several times after that but, as always, I was soon fit enough to be able to carry on my fight. I think that was the 'one step back'!!

I could not wash my hair for the seven months that my 'wires' were inserted and, with a very itching head, it was great wonder that I did not dislodge them by scratching. However, when I had my head dressed (re-bandaged) by the nurses they could see where my wires were inserted and also where they could scratch, and this was heaven. I dare not look at my wires. They had to work and I was entirely in the doctors' and nurses' hands and, needless to say, these were very traumatic times for me.

When I had had the wires in for two to three months I was allowed home for odd days, progressing to weekends and later for several days at a time as the time wore on. I went home armed with my 'box on my head' dressing and a headscarf to cover this monstrosity. I did not think of what everybody thought of me but I seemed to be accepted by friends and family as normal. Of course, normal it was not and they seemed not to understand just what was going one with me and even my husband seemed unconcerned.

I had good times and bad times and when it was bad the ward sister would repeat the saying 'two steps forward one step back', which was comforting at the time although with hindsight I did not think that I could possibly undergo this treatment again. But the words were comforting and my ongoing 'lifeline'; I knew that I had to persevere with my fight.

Before having surgery I was taking twelve

milligrammes of Neulactil tranquilizers. After surgery, I was reduced to six milligrammes and that meant that I would not be drowsy and could live a reasonably normal life; I must say that this seemed to be great improvement!!! To try to help me with my increasing anxiety, OCD and mood swings and child phobias, Dr Crow also prescribed lithium. At the time I was so impatient to have the wires out and to try and live a near normal life that I did everything I was told to do and was very grateful for the nursing and consultancy that I received.

After I had the wires in for seven months, I was perceived by the powers that be that my treatment had been sufficient and they removed them from my head. Apparently, the wires were in the same position when I had them removed as when they were inserted. It took five and a half hours for the electrodes to be inserted and about fifteen minutes to remove them. I had not had my hair washed for seven months so it was washed and set by a nurse and, when I had put on t he new dress that I had made previously, I was transformed!! It was a very traumatic experience and I have no wish to experience that episode again!

When I was discharged from the Burden Neurological Institute I experienced a sudden state of depression and was convinced that the surgery was unsuccessful but I think in hindsight that the success was 50/50 as Dr. Crow had informed me. I know that if I had not undertaken this surgery I would surely be no more now (in life).

Of course, now I have large dents in my head where the wires were inserted but this is a very small price to pay for saving my life. When I go to the hairdressers I am very aware of these dents but there is no going back again. It happened and I must accept this, which of course, I do.

By the way, before I had surgery and I had several EEGS (brain readings) and when I had had the wires in for seven months, I had another test to check that I had sustained sufficient treatment for the obsessive compulsive disorder and it seemed that I had had sufficient so they were removed!

Chapter 5 - Life after Surgery

Before I was admitted to the Burden Neurological Institute I had a very good job as a typist for Wiltshire County Council, but I lost this because of my second nervous breakdown and because I was deemed to be unreliable. Since the operation I have had several jobs and some of them have been extremely good, including one of the tax office in Bath. I have also managed to cope with several legal jobs, including audio positions, driven by desire to succeed and earn money. After I was married in 1966 I attained a Level II in City and Guilds in Literacy, gained several qualifications in shorthand, typing and English language. Later, after a course at Salisbury College I received Units I and II in Adult Learner Supported exams, but failed Unit III very badly and was ill after that. It was such a blow to my pride. I always want to learn and seem to have a very enquiring mind but my brain and it seemed my body was saying 'no'.

When I was married and worked as a clerical assistant at the Ministry of Defence I volunteered my notice, as I was then taking sixty milligrammes of Neulactil and kept falling asleep at work. Later, I had a job as a shorthand typist and was then promoted to secretary to a Major Spence, a senior member of the staff. While this was happening I took exams to enhance my education and attained qualifications in Shorthand and Typing. I then left General Accident and joined Pepler Jenkins, Solicitors, to work as a legal secretary, but I left because the money was too poor and went elsewhere. But this had started my legal career, which I found fascinating. Some time later, Mr. Jenkins of Pepler & Jenkins called round at my house and asked me to be his secretary. As this was music to my ears, I accepted. I loved working for the legal profession, found it interesting and challenging and enjoyed the comradeship within it. I was expected to make decisions on my own, and enjoyed this responsibility of this career very much.

My husband and lived in rented accommodation during this time until I began looking for a house, but my husband said that he did not want a mortgage round his neck!! After I had persuaded him that the mortgage would be no more than the rent we were now paying, he agreed to purchase our own house. We acquired the house and this was indeed my great sanctuary!! Although he was not really interested in it - as long as he had a pint of beer he was happy, that was enough for him.

When, some time later, my father-in-law died of lung cancer at the age of seventy, and I perceive that this was all due to his children and grandchildren worries, Angus's family seemed to fall apart and seemed uncoordinated without him, he was their bindweed so it seemed.

Well, it was not long before my mother-in-law stated that she could no longer live on her own, even though she had her family around her. Well, because of this pressure on us, we had to sell up to go and live with her, but she did not realise what this had done to me. My house was my haven, plus the work I had done in order to attain it - I was broken hearted!!! I think that Angus realised this later, but too late, and, as it seems to me with all sons, I felt his mother came first and that was when our marriage began to slide downhill.

I searched for comfort with other men. My life had been fractured and, as per usual, this was a mother-in-law I could not live with. She used to run after Angus and ignore me although I would work two jobs to his one and I felt ostracised. It was then that began to distance myself from the family, I was a little cog in a large wheel and because I did not fit very well, I felt disorientated and, again, very isolated. I had no friends because I could not communicate very well with people as my illness kept me apart from attaining this friendship.

While was married to Angus, amounting to a total of twenty-five years, I did not really get on with my in-laws. My life became a parody of swings and roundabouts in the extreme and I firmly now believe that what goes up must come down. I tried to gain my in-laws favour, and must have succeeded a bit as they did say at one time that I was one of the girls, but as they had their own children and consequently the grandchildren, my presence amounted to less than the others. I must admit that I was a little jealous of them and I craved their approval. I just thought that my husband loved me but I was a little disconcerted by his incessant drinking and then I became increasingly lonely and isolated.

Charlotte Harris

C'est la guerre!!!

Chapter 6 - My Second Marriage

When I met Ian in 1990, I was willing to be courted by him. I thought this was another affair, although I was definitely drawn towards him. He had arrived back from Africa, where he had been living for twenty years, to be with his family. He had a broken family background and also had a son who his wife would not allow him to see after their divorce. He was broken willed and down-hearted, but it is true to say that we had a deep understanding of each other and were well-suited. This was about the time I was beginning the menopause (at the age of forty-six). I was trying to get work in Bath but was not in very good health. I was still living with my husband, but matters were very disjointed. So, I would leave the mobile home (which we purchased when I persuaded Angus to leave his mother), catch the bus to work, see Ian where he worked and then return home to Angus.

However, about this time when Ian was working, he developed pneumonia (which he had suffered from before having weak lungs and suffering from asthma). So this time I would leave home, go to work and then go up to the Royal United Hospital in Bath to see Ian and then go home to my husband afterwards. It was something that I had to do, maybe a little silly but this was the basis of a strong relationship with Ian and I wanted to hang on to what I had got and, of course, eventually it led to true love and care.

I confided in Ian about my illness and he

confidentially told that I would be O.K. by the time I was fifty years old! What confidence! Little did he know of the life he was going to have with me afterwards. But his heart was all there.

Then came the menopause, and my hormones were all over the place, I had yet another nervous breakdown. Nonetheless, I now realised I had found the love of my life at forty-seven years old. The following months Ian and I shared intimacies about our lives and my illness. He was very caring and, through his deep love for me, came to have an understanding of what I was going through where no-one else had achieved this.

When I met Ian my cash control was a little out of hand (I had a credit card that was owed money) so he sorted this out for me. I also forgot my appointments with my psychiatrist Dr. Bird and was really quite ill. Ian made contact with Dr Bird, who then made an appointment to see me, with regular appointments thereafter so that was very satisfactorily accomplished. It just proves the state of mind I was in when I was with Angus; I had completely lost the plot! My life was uncoordinated and my own health was suffering.

In fact I was a bit of a wreck when I met Ian. He had to organise my life again from scratch. Soon I had Dr. Bird and the love of Ian, which became a good platform to start to build my new life again and that is just what I did.

So that is how Ian and I started together originally.

AN ABANDONED MIND

He had my welfare at heart and I warmed to his care and love for me, the like of which I had not experienced in my life prior to this date.

That was 1990 and all this time, I was living a triple life with two men, Angus and Ian. Ian had a broken heart because of the fact that his wife had divorced him and would not allow him to see is son. Things in Africa were becoming confrontational for him and he could see the signs that the country was breaking out of control against the white population. He had made a good fortune there, but he had paid for his wife to have her baby in England (necessary because she had gynaecological problems), which cost him his job. So he was broke when he came back to this country to be with his father, stepmother and brother.

After Ian and I had been seeing each other for some time, then came the words 'shall we go and live together'. By that time I had next to no life with Angus and I did not hesitate to say 'yes'.

I think Angus knew that there was something in the offing, after all we had been together for nearly twenty-five years. Well, we still had many rows and at one time he said to me 'why don't you f*** off'. Well I promptly said I would and then Angus broke down in tears and cried until the taxi had picked me up from the mobile home to take me off to be with Ian. When I left Angus I felt very sorry for him and whenever I rang him he would howl in tears. So I went back to him temporarily but I yearned for Ian so much that one night when Angus was working, I arranged to go back to Ian for good. Ian had entered the mobile home previously and the dog seemed not to mind him. Of course, it was sad that I would never see Cassie the dog again. But that's life and I had my love...

I arrived in a café in Bath where Ian and I had arranged to meet with my case and he seemed so relieved to see me in one piece, even though I was rather upset, what a wrench!!

Ian and I have now been together eighteen years and married ten years. But this time the difference is that I am happy and fulfilled. He is my full-time carer and it is a fact that in no way could I live without him now, even though looking after me is a mammoth task, and he knows it but would lay down his life for me.

At this time I was increasingly emotionally disturbed as I was severing at twenty-five year relationship but it was now on the cards as being done and finalised. This was the start of our life together and we decided to go to France to celebrate the break-up with Angus and my now new relationship and alliance with Ian.

Then came my next nervous breakdown. With hindsight I can see it was a mistake to go to France as I quite ill, but I managed to survive without medical care with the new love of my life. When we came back from France and lived in Salisbury, I would ring Angus and he would be crying desperately. I think I broke his heart but he has said since that he has great respect for Ian in maintaining his love and care for me.

At one time I felt so sorry for Angus, that I went back to him for a few days but as I longed for Ian so much that Angus was working nights, I stoked up t he fire for the dog and slipped away at night! Ian said that I had betrayed his love for me but because of that great love, he took me back and I never left his side again.

I was very sorry for Angus, as it was coming up to our twenty-fifth Wedding Anniversary, but through al the ups and downs, Ian was my man now and a much better life was waiting for me now

At this time I was in my forty-seventh year and began to commence the menopause. As if I did not have enough on my plate. Ian was caring and understanding and, as he had so much to offer and we also had much to offer each other, we gelled completely and this was real love at last!!!!! Ian wanted to know all about me, with sympathy, but we had no money and times were hard. We lived in a hotel temporarily and I would do some ironing for the owners to get a little money to help us.

By the time I was in my fifties Ian had spent an awful lot of money on me so that I would not brood. But my illness never waned and, as usual, I still had my breakdowns but they were now interspersed with deep love and understanding from Ian and we pulled through and whenever I became agitated if we were going away I would become unreasonable and our holiday would be ruined (by me)!

When we had been together for about seven years we had been going to see Ian's mother who was in a nursing home suffering from osteoporosis. She gave me her first engagement ring as a sign of her affection for me and intimated to us that she would like us to get married so that she could pass her son over to me. We were married in Salisbury in the Registry Office with much more minimal fuss than both our first marriages. We then took a photograph of us at the wedding to show to 'mother' and she was delighted.

A few months later she died but I firmly believe that maybe her prayer has now been answered. Of course, she did not know of my illness, and would not have been able to understand any of it, as it was so complicated. Anyway when Ian saw her in the 'chapel of rest' he found that in her hands were clutched the photos of our wedding so that made him feel more at ease. Of course it was terrible to lose his mother, and I now realised that she was my only friend in life. It is a pity that I had not shown her more love when she was alive but my love is with her now! I have her son so now she can rest in peace. I can now thank her for her mercy and for allowing me the greatest love of her life, her son.

Before Ian and I were married, I said to first my husband 'can we get divorced?' and he said 'I thought we were already divorced'. So that was then settled and I underwent proceedings with a solicitor to acquire this divorce as a mutual separation. Ian and I thought this was the best and easiest thing to do under the circumstances but, of course, at this time we did not know of Ian mother's demise. This hurt my husband greatly as he never knew that anyone could live with me in my state! In a way he was relieved about the divorce and he admired Ian for what he had taken on.

Angus is still alive but a hopeless alcoholic and, of course, the drink has damaged his brain irreversibly. He will still ring me now and talk about past events insinuating that the times we had together were good but there was always an edge to everything as I will relate later. We were soon swallowed up with unhappiness as time went on and he gave me a certain amount of love but definitely no understanding of what I went through in all those years. And that applies to his family as well. I think the right phrase is 'ignorance is bliss'! We were together for twenty-five years and I was too ill to make a break and he must have known that. We grew further and further apart.

When Ian came along, it was a pleasant awakening for me. He was my 'knight in shining armour' and also my saviour. We both had a past in common and intertwined immediately. We had a risky courtship for so many reasons but our relationship became 'rock solid'! As Ian put it 'we were a couple of golden oldies' and I would like to reiterate that for me love was definitely better the second time around. You just have to know what to look for and try and not make the same mistakes twice. Ian and

I were married in 1997 so that is over ten years ago.

One of the best and moving things Ian did for me was to establish me with the benefit Disability Living Allowance'. His first request was turned down, but following a tribunal he was successful, as he described that I had a cocktail of nervous illnesses and that I had also undergone a 'selective leucotomy'. My life had been a series of swings and roundabouts and I had never been able to hold a job down because of this ailment, only in short bursts, and this was very debilitating. My illness had encompassed me all my life and the suffering had been enormous. I had showed signs of discomfort in my early life and this had culminated in these many illnesses that I was unable to control. I had been abandoned by everyone that was close to me but Ian decided the best thing he could do was to attain this allowance for me so he went at it 'all guns blazing' and with Dr. Bird's (the Burden Neurological Institute) help including written proof of my illness, it was achieved.

I had six months back pay, but when you come to think of it, it was something I had needed all my life, I just needed that little bit of love and care that Ian gives me, and I shall be grateful to him and always love him for that.

Chapter 7 - Looking Back and Reflecting

If I stand back and view my first marriage I think it could best be summarised as follows:

Before and during my first marriage I embarked on a career as a legal secretary. I found the law a fascinating occupation with its matrimonial, conveyancing and probate sides. I enjoyed the responsibility, when the boss was away from the office, seeing clients and making decisions in his absence. I worked for a solicitor twice in Bath, on the second occasion when I was asked back to a company by the senior partner in order to be his secretary. Later on I worked in Bristol as a legal audio typist 'temp' for three years but found the fulltime employment and the travelling too much. I loved my interaction between lawyer and Counsel and once when I was working in Bath; my boss invited me to the Court to see him win his case!!

Of course, when I was a legal secretary there was a lot of 'engrossing' to perform on all the Deeds so there had to be no errors on the engrossment parchment. I think that it may be a little different now with clauses file on a 'computer' and it is probably much simpler now but I enjoyed the old way and I was often to witness a document while I was employed by the Solicitors. Legal Secretarial work was very popular with even some shorthand thrown in as well, if called for so one had to be reasonably adaptable. For this short time, I could do something that I was trained for but when I had to give up fulltime employment at the age of thirty five, the choices were not so numerous.

Now to my first marriage: my mother-in-law had a rough time in the war, bringing up her family. She cried a lot and suffered epileptic fits (although I did not witness one of these). The doctors put her on Phenobarbitone tablets and, when I was so ill, she said that I should take these as they were wonderful for her. Of course, she did not know my problems and I suppose she was only trying to be helpful. I am afraid that I could not accept her advice about what I should do about my health, she was not aware of my symptoms!! Anyway, she coped with her illness, as I did mine, but we were oceans apart!!

During my treatment at the Burden Neurological Institute and my subsequent attempt at suicide and during the trips to my home wearing a headscarf, my husband stood by me and visited regularly. I was not the perfect wife. Dr. Crow had not asked to see him but he knew from Dr. Smythe all about me. But Dr. Crow's target was my 'little grey cells' but, he did not see me when I had the wires in and I remember a Sister at the Burden telling me that the treatment would act as 'two steps forward and one step back'. Of course, she was right but even when I was discharged after seven months; I was still not convinced it had worked.

My foster parents never came near me when I was in the Burden Neurological Institute. They did not agree that I should have brain surgery and showed it that way; it was quite beyond them and they did not know that if it had not been for the operation I would not have survived in life. It was a feeling of isolation, not knowing what was around the corner but it was certain that it had saved my life. Angus said that the operation had changed my personality but nobody seems to know whether for good or bad!!!!

It was a very traumatic experience!!

My husband Angus humiliated me in many things that I did, like throwing a ball to the in-laws' children. I do not have good co-ordination due, I believe, to my genes. Actually the worst thing he did to me was that he could not accept the fact that I would not stay in a job for long. He sympathised but was never surprised. He knew that I was good at my work but would not investigate why this should happen. He just seemed to accept it and did not want to take it any further. It became a big joke to him and this was why he said I should be in the 'Guinness Book of Records', because of the number of jobs I had had. He would tell other people as well and this was his big joke against me.

I did not get on very well with people and we had no friends except his drinking friends of which I was no part. We used to go off on day trips in the car with the in-laws and, after he had introduced his father to a drink, it would be a pub crawl all the way home. It made me very frustrated as I usually had to go to work the next day and this, of course, was my priority. He would not relish buying me a 'coffee' as I could not drink alcohol and he ostracised me for this.

As Angus worked in a factory, his language became suspect, and every other word seemed to be the 'f' word, but his family seemed to accept this and the affection between him and his mother was very noticeable as I learnt to my cost later on.

When we sold our home in Victoria Buildings, in order to care for mother-in-law, we managed to make a little money from the sale of the house, but we had to forego about two thousand pounds due to the expenses of living and needing to complete certain repairs. This left us with fifteen thousand pounds as a clean result of our sale. Many rows occurred at the Grove and, although we had a sink in our room, we could never really be independent of the mother-in-law. Time went on and I became increasingly unhappy with my living conditions. Tempers would fly with the family and I eventually decided that I could stand this no more. I heard of a mobile home in Box, in Wiltshire for sale for eleven thousand pounds,

Against my husband's wishes we bought it and moved to our new home!!! Angus said it hurt him greatly to sever the ties with his mother, but I needed some sanity and, after all she had three more daughters who could quite easily share the responsibility of looking after her. Of course she was getting old and as with all old women it is the son that they cannot lose. Anyway, she did not lose him but they both lost me!!! Angus said that he hated the mobile home but when I left him in 1989 he said he would not live anywhere else. He seemed to be a real 'turncoat'.

AN ABANDONED MIND

When I was married to Angus, I still had no security or understanding that I could speak of so I had affairs in order t o try and find happiness. I did not seem to be short of suitors and secrecy was essential on both sides, (my lover and I) as my suitors were also married and this had to be a sworn secret on either side. Angus and I grew further apart, due to his excessive drinking and, when he had bronchitis, which was quite often he would go to the doctor and get antibiotics. We all know that antibiotics will make you feel better after a few days, so he would then leave them off in order to take a drink. I think that most of the time the drink saturated the symptoms and that is how he continued.

My life (until I met Ian) seemed to be a life of aspirations and dreams, most of them unattainable. People have said to me in the past, 'do this' or 'do that and all will be well' but this never happened. I have had to blind myself to life and carry on as best I can and my experiences have been a diary of mixed emotions, which, no matter how hard I try come to me in the often disturbing dreams. I am sure one's memories are intact through life and they will seem to come back and haunt one. I suppose that is what we have a memory for. Most dreams seem to be difficult to cope with as they seem to be like jigsaws, even then, they cannot be denied. But my dreams are a bible of my past life and come to me in a variety of transparent voids. My life has been quite full, and I have many of these memories which, I fear, I can never destroy.

I think, with hindsight, that it was impossible to improve the situation as in my first marriage I did not have the understanding and guidance that Ian now gives me. It really was a 'comedy of errors' and there was no real way out. I seemed then to be naïve about life, with little common sense, which seemed to hinder my progress. When Angus did not work for a year I think he must have had a conscience about my working full time (and yet not succeeding). Tempers would flair and it was a very traumatic experience for both of us. I eventually found out that he had become a full-time drinker and later applied at the University of Bath for a security guard position. He attained this (to my relief) but it involved working shift work, including nights. He would come home in the morning and get into bed. I would take the dog out, and then go to work. Of course, this sort of habit really ruins a marriage and I found myself living a double life. When my husband was sleeping in the day I found I was very upset by the noises of the children next door and this would upset me greatly. The other neighbours were not up to much and I found myself shouting at them because I was only trying to protect his necessary sleep.

About 1967 being married and still working at the Ministry of Defence in Bath, I became pregnant, but only realised this when I was told by friends in the toilet where we all used to meet and gossip that I had miscarried. It was then that I went on the 'pill'. I do not think that my husband knew about this but I think I did the right thing at the time. At the time Angus expressed his desire not to have children so it was just as well. I do not think that he was, at that moment, responsible to be a father. But I became broody later. I remember asking Dr, Crow if it would be a good idea to start a family but he just said 'I would not advise it'. He had saved my life again!!

People said that when I got married and had children of my own, the illness would go but I knew this was an old wives' tale and realised that there would be no cure for me at all. In fact, when I was married I was stepping out of the frying pan into the fire. Time was going to tell me that, but I was naïve and also in love initially and this sure was a learning curve!

I also now understand that you never know anyone until you live with them!!

A few years after I was married I was admitted to the Royal United Hospital in Bath with a hiatus hernia. For months I had been continually sick when vertically opposed and, when we went on holiday for a week I had to take a bucket for the nights. I could not eat any acid like tomatoes, as I would choke and throw up.

Anyway, I was on a large amount of drugs and the hospital said I would have to come off these in order to absorb the anaesthetic so I had to cease them. However, I became very ill because I was not taking the drugs as usual and the hernia was getting worse. I would just lie down and be immediately sick. Eventually I had the operation, and then went for Forbes Fraser Hospital in Bath to convalesce. I remember it very well as it was January and we were having thunderstorms.

My foster parents came to see me in hospital but I was so young and raring to go they did not see me very debilitated! The hospital made a bit of a mess of my stomach but I was so relieved to be normal again. After all, who was going to see my scars. I definitely had more of those to come! I think, because of my drug situation and the imminent need of the surgery, it was maybe rushed a little. Since then, apart from continual hiccups, I have faired well. This was the first of my major operations and there were two more to come!!

When Angus and I were in our second flat, we were told we could have no children. The owners lived above us and promptly had a baby. This did not go down very well with me, as there was noise overhead and at this time I yearned for my own house and was becoming 'broody'. I worked at the Gas Board and, as I was paid for the amount of work I did in the time stipulated, I tried to earn a deposit for a house of our own!!

It was at this time that I had anther breakdown (overwork) and this was mainly depressive and I was admitted to Weston Lodge Hospital Psychiatric Unit in Bath. I could not stop crying and even though Angus bought a new car to hopefully cheer me up, this did not transpire. During my life I have endured sixteen ECT treatments but always seemed to come round crying profusely!!

AN ABANDONED MIND

I realised, that after several treatments, nothing seemed to be being achieved so I discharged myself and ran back to 'The Grove' where my in-laws lived and also my husband. I stayed there for some time but still yearned for a place of my own. My father-in-law encouraged this. He had a soft spot for me, I carried on working and we soon had the deposit for a house. Angus was not all that keen about a mortgage but we eventually bought a house of our own. I made the home my own, with curtains and accessories and we often had family in to our house to stay. I do not think that Angus was happy there as he would spend no money on the house. I still worked full time and we would often go out with the family.

We acquired a dog while living in our house and this was our first pleasure and we enjoyed this company and went out with it often. We had the dog for only a few years, but then its liver gave out and we had to put it down which broke both our hearts. Now, while we were living in the house, my father-in-law made advances to me, which I found to be repulsive - he kissed me and could not understand why I did not respond. I cannot seem to think what he thought of his son!!! We were in the house several years but I was unwell and kept going down to Angus's work, around the corner, crying my eyes out and making a spectacle of myself. He had lived with me for some time now yet did not know my suffering.

It was while we were in the house that my husband would not go to work on a Monday morning (usually because of a weekend hangover) and we would go off to the coast, if I had a day off. He would make sure that all his workmates had gone to work, which was around the corner of our road at the local Stothert and Pitt factory and then we would go off. Now this day was quite fun but I knew I had to ring in his 'work' on his behalf and lie that he was sick. Sometimes, on the Tuesday, he would not want to go into work again, so the same thing happened. I am afraid that Angus liked to drink too much and our whole lives were punctuated with these sorts of happenings and this gradually undermined our marriage. I did still love my husband very much and I believe that he loved me but he would not understand my illness and could not see the gravity of what he had taken on. His family were also naïve and did not understand me.

I went from job to job but each one was terminated by my poor health. I would work all week then spent all the weekend doing the housework. When I later did some 'temp' legal work in Bristol, by the time I arrived home it was time to cook, wash up and go to bed, then it was up early the next day for early start Bristol. This went on for about three years.

When I was living with mother-in-law, this really was a no-go area for me. At the start of this time my husband would not work properly and there were many rows between myself and my in-laws and it was then that I decided I could not go on living with my mother-in-law, hence the purchase of the mobile home which we bought with the proceeds of our house. I am afraid that this was just a disaster waiting to happen. Other people must have this problem but at least we had a little money and could be on our own once more. At this time I started with two jobs and mother-in-law said she admired me for this but seemed not to convey this momentum to Angus, I know that work for me was a sort of obsession but I was just trying to survive, and secretly desiring an independent life for myself. I felt isolated and insignificant, like a tiny scarlet pimpernel flower amongst poppies in a cornfield.

When I was in my mid-thirties it was discovered that I had cervical cancer and that my smear tests had been very doubtful and I had to keep having them 'double checked'. After a check up some several years later I was again in surgery but after the surgery I when I left the operating theatre, I haemorrhaged and it was a rush to the operating theatre to be stitched up again. I then had to have my cervix stretched and, after that, my sex life waned and by the mid forties, my sex life was over. I think that my cervical cancer was so severe that I had to have nearly all the cells removed. I seemed to be lurching from one disaster to another!! I also thought that this contributed to my early menopause!!!

In September, 2003, when I was sixty years old I had a penchant for learning so enrolled myself on a Course at Salisbury College for an Adult Learner Support course, designed to teach the skills to help young people with learning difficulties in the English

Language. It was in three units and Unit I was very technical in which I typed and submitted the various examination questions and passed eventually.

Unit II was a course in the classroom helping students with their writing and grammar. After this I typed a long list of questions about the students, listening to their problems and some of them passed City and Guilds Literacy I in literacy and computer work. I felt that I actually had a place there and that I was doing some good for these students. I spent much time with my tutor before and after each session and learned many important points that would improve my chances of passing this exam.

This course took about a year to complete and I really had the 'teaching bug'. Any way I also passed Unit II and felt that my brain had been aired thoroughly well to all intents and purposes. I have now these two certificates at home on the lounge wall together with my Literacy II'

But by the time I came to Unit III the pressure had got to me and, of course, my illness, which is not really an excuse as I did not have the required ability, and failed this unit. Well, that was my volunteer teaching out the window!! I was then ill again which was only expected to happen and I felt very let down by the system. I was very hyper about this exam and I think that I bit off more than I could chew. Well, it certainly was a learning curve and I attained this at the age of sixty. I also learnt about computers as of course when I achieved my

AN ABANDONED MIND

RSA III this was on a manual typewriter.

I do not know if these things will be of any use to me in the future but I have gleaned an awful lot with these activities and they are all stored in my brain!!!!.

Chapter 8 - Ongoing Anxieties

In my darkest hour I feel ill and have a sense of foreboding; no matter how hard I try, nothing seems to go right for me, I have never been blessed with any luck, and even God seems to have forsaken me. I feel that I was an unwanted child and because I was weak, then perhaps it would have been better if I had not been born. Do you feel like this at times? Well, I can tell you there is an answer. I know Hitler would have got rid of me; I was one of the weak ones and therefore did not deserve to survive - only the strongest ones did.

I cannot live without my drugs; they are my lifeline and have been since I was aged sixteen years. I think somehow that the illness could be 'gene generated'. My family, three brothers and three sisters all seemed to be affected in some way. My sister has recently died of Huntington's Chorea, the illness that my mother also died of!!

Anyway, thanks to other people in my life, I have managed to survive, but I know this illness will haunt me all my life!!! This is a story for others in a similar position, to say that resilience is essential and that life has had its rewards. But the greatest thing I have now is love and understanding from my now second husband, which I think is an essential contribution and this will help along the way. There must be no place for fear, for that, of course, is what this illness is all about. It is a tremendous battle, but as is often said 'don't let the bastards get you down' because, believe me, as you know, they will if they can.   Don't let them win and it will be your salvation and then you will always be able to empathise with others of your experience in life!!

Child Phobia

It is at times like this that I wish I was not here. My ears prick to children's talk, and if there is one child there I see a dozen. The sight of a child's summer dress, or appropriate, sends shiver down my spine. Among the sights and signs I hear there are more discharged in my vivid imagination. I get very angry, what rights have they to be there (I think) making me oh so aware of my torture'. My hearing is so acute and even sounds that are quite normal, sound like children to me. When I see the children, I can assess nervously their noise, but when I do not see them, it is like a thunderbolt and find myself shaking violently.

I can put myself into a prepared position and cope reasonably well. When children's noises come out of the blue then I seem to be filled with fear, it upsets me so much that it can often take me a hour or two to calm down. I do not have any personal feelings against children. I just fear what this sound will do to me and my resultant reactions. This, it seems is a phobia - a most unpleasant one, I fear!!!

When I am alone, and even when Ian and I are together, children alarm me very much and I do not wish them to be near me, for fear!! I can hear them a mile away and face with great fear the school holidays, which I suppose is rather obvious and it does not seem to matter what the ages of the children are.

I am afraid that at our site we have had much

trouble, especially with neighbour's grand children involving the Police and we have even had damage to our property because of a father's reaction. This is an uncontrollable fear and anxiety for me!!!

I have undertaken Cognitive Behavioural Therapy, but although there was temporary relief, it was not permanent as the anxieties seem to be ingrained into me and I have to work around it rather then shake it off.

My husband protects me well against children and we try to avoid them if possible, but of course, sometimes it is not. When the neighbour's grandchildren upset me I find it very hard to control my feelings, (mostly anger) and my husband always seems to get the brunt of it. Of course, this means that I do not get on with my neighbours, but there seems to be no 'quick fix', so I try my best to get on with them as best I can and hope for the best. Of course, it is nothing personal to do with them and not their fault but this is how it is.

Although we have had a new soundproofed door fitted to the front, we also have had triple glazing put in the windows in the front. I always have the curtains drawn in the lounge, with hardly any sight and sound except for my own television sound and music that I play on the CD. I am also very sensitive to other noises, people's voice, and banging and lawn-mowing of any kind.

I have no confidence in myself and feel that I am being persecuted by everyone and I also feel that children are going to attack me, this making me feel very threatened and stressed. I get very angry and have to move away from these situations and I fear and get nightmares about my impending predicaments. I am jealous and resentful and at odds with other people as they all seem to pose a threat but I now that this is only in my own mind but it is very difficult to keep it there, contained.

All my OCD, panic attacks, phobias and manic depression are summed up in one word – horrific! I always said that this was mental torture but in my mood swings I have 'up' and 'downs' and I find myself praying for an 'up' to relieve my anxiety. I fear everything and everybody, but this is all in my brain and is a threat to my sanity, I fear. Life is very difficult for me but I am lucky in having a man who loves me and understands. True carers are very rare and to have someone who cares and someone that I also love is absolutely vital!

Dr. Crow from the Burden Neurological Institute once told me that 'all nervous illnesses are born of fear' and, to this day I am sure that his words were sacrosanct!! Colour seems like people, even children, to me. I also see shapes that my mind puts into the shape of children. Such is my fear! To illustrate how this plays on my imagination, I have, at times, heard noises that sound like children, and I have sent my husband outside who reports that there is no-one there. It seems to me that voices, sounds seem to irritate me, it is peace I long for away from this persecution above all, peace of mind!!

AN ABANDONED MIND

This is a weary road I walk, full of chastisement and criticism of myself. I wonder why I persevere, but I know that there is a light at the end of the tunnel and I always remember the sister telling from the Burden Neurological Institute telling me 'two steps forward, one step back' and I live my life by this creed. It is not easy but I feel I may be able to help someone else along the way by relating this experience. After all, I am sixty four years of age now and still alive and I now have my husband, the love of my life, and who is my fulltime carer, even though I had to wait until I was forty six years old to have my life resuscitated. It was definitely worth the wait, but, under different circumstances I may not have been here to tell the story.

There is, and always will be a stigma attached to this illness and, although all my life I have hidden these symptoms to assume 'normality' my heart goes out to those who suffer similarly and they are definitely not mad, but emotionally disturbed, which is completely different. One way or another you can say we are over-sensitive to others and, when in life or institution we all have many stories to tell, and are definitely not alone. We become more tolerant and understanding of others' emotions. Yet, I will say that through my life experiences I have become very bitter, which is a sin!

Things in life have to be thought over to try and contain one's anger. God knows, I seem to have enough of that, I have a temper that has to be quelled by talk and reasoning. I think that my illness undermines this very often and I have to simmer down, but, of course, I have my wonderful husband now and I know he is always there for me.

There is no 'quick fix', one has to go through the tunnel before seeing the light at the end, and this is one of the most difficult things to do! But we can all arrive there in the end, and we are more mature people for our suffering.

AN ABANDONED MIND

THIS IS THE STORY OF LIVING WITH EXTREME ANXIETY, OR, as I would say 'LIVING WITH AN ABANDONED MIND'

I do not think that many people have experienced a similar life to mine of depression. OCD, anxiety and phobias, and have gone through brain surgery as a result of this. These seem to all be in extreme degrees.

This is the story of my life, from orphaned beginnings to foster care (of abuse) and a marriage of twenty five years. The reason that I call it abandoned is that no-one during my early years could understand my illness and I was destined to a marriage of twenty-five years with no understanding and a make-believe 'love'. They all seemed to turn a blind eye to it; it seemed too complicated for them to understand, so they just ignored it|!

It was not until my later years and a second marriage that I achieved it. Then I had to hide all my real feelings and impulses and I underwent brain surgery (at that time I was a guinea pig) and apart from the surgery saving my life there does not seem to be any cure.

I hope this script will help those with one or more of these feelings and emotional disturbances and encourage these people to fight on.

There is a light at the end of the tunnel. You are not alone and I am telling you this story at the age of sixty four years. There is no such thing as 'giving up' or having to accept an end.

OCD

From a very early age I had the compulsion to touch things unnecessarily. Later on in my life I found that all lines, gaps, angles and dots had to be touched and also I wanted to close all gaps and spaces but of course I did not do this physically so I would feel senses in my fingers and various other parts of my body. If I was watching television watching someone put on a coat then I would feel this sensation of myself putting on the coat. Also, if a car is driving over a line and there would be spaces between the bottom of the car and the lines. I will purse my lips in order to satisfy my nerve sensor.

Of course, I grind my teeth as well, to satisfy my needs and the nerves all over my body respond to these completions.

When you come to think of it, everything is a line, a corner, an angle, dot or spaces to my whole body is a mass of nerve discomfort.

This is a very crippling disorder which I believe to be some kind of obsessional neurosis, and this also applies to gaps in sounds, raindrops on the window or elsewhere allowing a gap between each drop - which I have also a compulsion to close. Another peculiar sensation I experience is having to turn away from sunlight flashing through trees for fear that something will happen to me. Also, when I am walking down stairs (with lines painted across them) I falter at the bottom few steps and lose my balance.   These seem an odd addition, but nevertheless, they are true and factual.

Chapter 9 - A Carers Perspective

Part 1

When adults attain the age of three score years and ten, they begin to reflect upon the highs and lows in their lives. When I do so, there are some devastating lows, but there are also some creditable highs. At the top of my list must be my apparent ability to care for the disabled.

My caring experience began at a very early age, when, at the age of around fifty one my mother had a complete nervous breakdown. The problems of bringing up a small boy in the height of World War II were too much for her. There was absolutely no help available and I was suffering from chronic asthma, which can be attributed to the near miss from the German bomb which damaged out house.

Anyway, when one is faced with severe crises it brings out the best in one. Mother's chief problem was lack of food. We had a small plot of land (about five yards by fifteen yards) at the back of our small flat and I set about growing some food. So here was a five or six years old growing vegetables (by trial and error I might add). Very soon the neighbours started to barter with me and I was in business.

When I was still pre-teen, I befriended a boy of similar age. He was a very serious case of haemophilia and his name was Alan King. His father was the local butcher and the area where we lived was near Penenden Heath on the outskirts of Maidstone in Kent.

Alan and I became friends and, as the years progressed we became inseparable. Alan's illnesses, for there were several, were very distressing and he spent many days bedridden. I used to go around and talk and play board games in his bedroom.

As time went by, Alan developed two great passions in his life. The first was stamp collecting and the other was train-spotting. I was to become seriously involved in both and even developed my own passion for these pastimes.

Many the time I can remember going into Maidstone on the bus with Alan, and spending our pocket money on stamps. Alan took great pride in his collection. I can even remember the name of the stamp shop. It was Potters in Week Street in Maidstone opposite the then offices of the local newspaper, The Kent Messenger.

As we both grew older we were allowed days out train spotting and also went to the Saturday morning films at the Granada Cinema in Maidstone.

Out train experiences started at Maidstone, Kent which was a very busy mainline rail junction and finally we even went to Clapham Junction East station; then we graduated to Ashford (Kent) outside Waterloo in London.

One of our greatest thrills was not so far afield. We used to travel, by bus, to Paddock Wood Station in the morning and watch the Golden Arrow thunder through at between ninety and one hundred miles an hour. Paddock Wood is halfway between Ashford and Tonbridge and the rail track is dead straight for about twenty miles. The Golden Arrow was nearly always hauled by a Battle of Britain class engine and that gave us an additional thrill as we were both very proud to have survived a battle in which we were spectators.

As a result of our travels Alan's legs grew stronger and we even ventured out onto the mini golf course on Penenden Heath. Because of his illness Alan developed a very competitive nature and I took up the challenge and, weather permitting, many hours were spent locked in battle on the mini golf course.

All throughout our travels I was never worried or even thought about the implication if Alan were to have an accident. I was blissfully unaware of the responsibilities which rested upon me. I suppose you could call it the ignorance of youth. Anyway, Alan's parents trusted me to get him home without accident and because I achieved this aim, you could say that the Gods of Good Fortune smiled upon me.

After my eleventh birthday I was sent away to boarding school, so my time with Alan was restricted to school holidays. I am pleased to relate that we simply increased our adventures to compensate for my absences!

AN ABANDONED MIND

I am still, to this day, very distressed to recall that this story did not have a happy ending.

By the time he was around sixteen or so, Alan was allowed a custom built tricycle. It had large wheels and served to strengthen his leg muscles.

When we were both eighteen years of age our ways divided; I finished school and went to do my two years National Service. Alan was broken hearted at my enforced absence. Later his parents told me he was inconsolable at my absence.

One day, I was told, it was very wet, windy and horrible. Alan rode his tricycle to the top of the steepest of the many hills in the area, then pedalled furiously down hill, straight into the front of a bus which was picking up passengers at the bottom of the hill.

I am told that, at the point of impact, he must have been travelling at, at least, forty miles per hour and death was instantaneous.

As you can well imagine Alan's parents were very distressed. I gradually drifted away from Maidstone as I set off on my travels to Africa and beyond.

However, fifty three years on I still think of Alan King. It just shows how, with help, the disabled can cope with their problems, but take that hope or help away and disaster can not be far away.

Part 2

To write this paper properly I find difficult. There are so many facets and every carer must face different problems, making accurate assessment almost impossible. Anyway, I have tried to put matters from my personal perspective and I hope the reader will make allowances.

By definition a carer is described as 'anyone who looks after someone who cannot manage at home without some support. This may be because of illness, disability mental health needs or learning difficulties'.

It is estimated that there are 40,000 carers in Wiltshire alone. All have different problems and circumstances.

In my case, my wife Charlotte (Lottie) has severe OCD coupled with episodes of depression and anxiety. By far the most important medical event in Charlotte's life has been her brain operation. In the early 1970s she underwent a serious operation in Frenchay Hospital in Bristol. The after effects lasted a full 7 months, during which time she was in the car of Dr. Harry Crow and his staff, at the Burden Neurological Institute. I will not elaborate on the details of the operation suffice it to say it was very complicated and Dr. Crow would not guarantee any real degree of success.

However, the success was enough to save Charlotte's life and give her some quality of life even to this day. We have lived together for eighteen years (married for ten) so I have developed a survival regime which suit both of us.

The main part of the operation (selective frontal leucotomy) involves burning part of the brain cells away using electric current. The operation was designed to block off part of the brain which was causing so much distress.

However, I have a theory that by means of love and care we are reopening the good parts of the brain which have been dormant for so long. In recent years I have noticed that Lottie has become so much more lucid. She has re-emerged as a typist of some stature and also she has mastered the basics of computing.

Where else can one find anyone who has survived this brain procedure and become so lucid? That is a plus and a testimony to what a carer can achieve.

To cope with these symptoms I have had to adapt to a totally different lifestyle and it has taken all of eighteen years to do so. I still find it difficult to put into accurate words, so please make allowances if the following appears disjointed and rambles. Perhaps this vague inability is the curse of a layman thrust into a caring role, which is the very nature of the animal that is our adversary.

The greatest sacrifice of all is to lay down your life for your friends and country.

I maintain that the second greatest sacrifice must be full time caring. Where else does the commitment require three hundred and sixty five days a year and twenty four hours a day on call? Although not physically ill, my wife's anxiety/depressions often border on suicidal tendencies hence the unrelenting commitment. The greatest compensation that I receive is the love of my wife who openly admits that she could not cope if I were in any way absent from her life. Prior to our meeting she tells me she has attempted suicide twice. I acknowledge that these attempts on her life might be 'cries for help' rather than the real thing, but all the while the threat remains one must be on one's guard ALL the time.

Sometimes when Lottie is seriously ill (as much as twice a year on average) I feel completely overwhelmed. It appears as an all consuming conflagration. Eventually it subsides and the aftermath is that I feel absolutely drained of energy and motivation for days afterwards. If I feel so drained after a bout of Lottie's illness I can only imagine the stress and commitment of carers who have to care for people with more physical needs such as dressing, washing and toilet etc.

People who are in authority who profess to appreciate carers' contributions do not, in my opinion, understand the problems fully. If they did they would increase the meagre remunerations given to carers. I am getting political and must move on. Before I do, I would add that one could write a complete paper on the shortcomings of help from a carer's viewpoint.

In particular I think the most important point is the withdrawal of National Health Service support following the recent reorganisation of the Health System. The lack of financial aid is written in stone but on the ground carers feel more neglected and vulnerable then ever.

To combat this detrimental change my wife and I have become much closer and we form a team to combat our problems. As a result we seem to be more relaxed about our plight. We have developed an 'us versus them' attitude and as a result we seem to be quite successful.

Recently, Lottie had a moderate intensity OCD attack and, with this paper in mind, I made a few notes and here they are:

First of all let me explain that in order to combat the worst excesses of Lottie's illness we have, together, agreed a code of conduct which differentiates certain areas which are forbidden.

Recently Lottie had an attack of OCD which was so severe that it took over her life completely and as a result she breached our self imposed code of conduct.

At the time Lottie knew she was doing wrong but the grip of the OCD on her mind was so strong that she was totally unable to say 'no'. This attack started when we were apart for an hour or so and by the time that we met the power of the obsession had begun to diminish. When Lottie told me what she had done, we had a huge row. My blood pressure went through the roof!!!

In these circumstances I have been taught to walk away for my own good and sanity. After a couple of hours of being separated and on our own, Lottie came to me as if nothing had happened. In other words the power of the obsessive attack had gone. The whole process took about three to four hours.

In the end Lottie then acts as if nothing has happened, but for me the damage to me is so great it takes me several days to recover.

I have been with Lottie for eighteen years, of which we will have been married for over ten years and every time her illness strikes in the intensity described, it takes me longer to recover. My ability to cope with sever attacks is weakening and what really worried me is what will happen in the end?

I have been having treatment for high blood pressure for the past five or six years. Also I have attended an anger management course and also a course run buy a lady psychiatrist on how to say 'no' without causing distress. However, my experience tells me, that however well a carer is prepared, they can never deal one hundred percent satisfactorily with a severe obsessive attack.

Attacks occur at the oddest times and without warning. I find that if a carer tries to anticipate an attack, then they never occur!!

To illustrate my point, in April 2007 Lottie wanted to go to the West End of London shopping. This is not an unusual request so I agreed. I do not mind admitting that I was scared out of my wits at the prospect of an illness attack.

There were rail problems at Waterloo so our journey Warminster to Waterloo involved two changes of train. To my amazement Lottie actually enjoyed the journey. Even the most experienced commuter would have flinched at the prospect. When we arrived at the West End I set up a system of mobile phone links in case of problems. We then separated for almost four or five hours.

You can imagine my astonishment when we met, there was a smiling happy Lottie absolutely weighted down with shopping. The return journey was just as difficult and, when we arrived home, the only thing Lottie complained about was tiredness.

This event proves to me that severe attacks which are OCD related can strike when they are least expected. Then, suddenly, bang, there they are. I have never discovered a common factor that can cause an attack. When they happen, I always get so frustrated that I accuse Lottie of betraying my trust in her, but when the dust settles, I realise it is the illness that has completely taken over her life/actions!!

On the other side of the coin I can illustrate

occasions when the illness has struck at funny and often serious or embarrassing moments. I can relate at least 4 occasions when illness has struck whilst we have been abroad:

1) At Bristol Airport upon return from a super holiday in Italy.
2) Remonstrating with a coach driver again in Italy when we had lost our way.
3) At a shopping arcade in Lille in France
4) On a sea trip to Bilbao in Spain.

Not all were on holiday. We have had serious problems in Bristol, Bath, and Bournemouth and I could go on for ages.

Do not get the impression that all this happens on holiday. Many attacks have occurred in and around home.

Some people may say that some of these incidents were physical and should be treated as such. I disagree; I know that there is something in her illness which prompts a brush with physical injury on top of the mental distress.

As a result of our experiences whilst travelling, we have now agreed not to go abroad and continue our holidays to local excursions.

Over the years we have tried many therapies to alleviate Lottie's symptoms, they include:

AN ABANDONED MIND

☐ Knitting
This is about the most successful therapy tried. I say this because Lottie keeps returning to it. However if she becomes too much involved in it, there could be a chance of triggering off the OCD attacks.

☐ Sewing
The same as above but overall Lottie is not too keen. And it is also a lost more expensive.

☐ Further Education
We have tried this over a two year period at Salisbury College. We did have some success exam-wise but it proved to be too expensive. Also, more importantly, her specialist warned Lottie that some subjects, Maths in particular, are conducive to the illness and Lottie was forced to abandon this therapy.

In recent years, Lottie has developed a very marked and serious phobia. She has developed a pathological hatred of children's noises. The distress ranges from any contact with age group of toddlers to early teens.

We tried to get treatment and eventually Lottie had a course of Cognitive Behavioural therapy at Red Gables, the local community mental health team base in Trowbridge. The course was administered by a nurse therapist. At the conclusion he wrote at length to say that the treatment had been successful, but I regret to write that I know it did not work. The fear of these sounds was so engrained in

Lottie's mind I mean.

The nurse therapist based his findings on set tasks which Lottie performed as instructed. The main drift of this treatment was confrontational. Lottie and I had to stand by a playground for as long as she could bear, or go into a crowded shopping mall.

The reason why this did not work was because Lottie's illness is triggered by the unexpected meeting with children or sudden exposure to their noise. Note the repeat of the dreaded words 'unexpected'. It is impossible to guard against, which makes the caring so exhaustive.

There is also one rather alarming aspect of this phobia. I reckon that I am reasonably stable and sane and I try to be the rock around which Lottie can cling; I now seem to have caught the phobia. I think possibly the reason may be that I am being over-protective.

I have tried my best to insulate Lottie from the constant contact with children and I am managing to get a new sound-proofed front door fitted, and our front windows are triple glazed. Despite these precautions Lottie insist that the front window curtains remain drawn day and night, rain or shine.

Caring for this phobia is very difficult. I try to steer her away from possible trouble spots when we are out. But the problem really arises when we are at home. As usual, it is the crisis which appears right out of the blue and unexpectedly. As a result we have very strained relations with nearly all our neighbours, as you cannot stop children visiting their relations!

One incident the problems got so bad that an irate parent caused criminal damage to our property. It took quite a while for the fallout to die down. Also we have had numerous visits from the police, both called by us and other parties.

Now you see why a carer has to acquire the skills of a seasoned diplomat. Not only these qualities, but also the carer has to be sympathetic, strong (both mentally and physically) as well as caring. What a job!!

My final submission is that the successful treatment of these mental illnesses can best be summed up as 'continuity and stability'.

Part 3 - A Carer's Appreciation of the Burden Neurological Institute

My wife was an inpatient for seven months in the early 1970's at the Burden Neurological Institute. She was also an outpatient, from that time until the move to Frenchay Hospital early in 2002. My involvement only started when early in the 1990's.

When we reflect upon the history of great British Medical Institutions one immediately ponders in terms of hundreds of years. Yet few institutions can have had such a dramatic influence on medical advancement then the Burden Neurological Institute has, in just a few short years. If it were possible to measure the volume of influence achieved per year of existence then the Burden Neurological Institute must feature high up in any league.

In sixty seven years the treatment of serious mental health has advanced almost beyond all recognition. Burden has been one of the driving forces in this advancement.

I can illustrate my comments. When my wife was eighteen she was admitted to the Roundway Mental Hospital in Devizes with severe depression and associated symptoms. She was told that there was nothing that could be done to help her so she discharged herself. As far as I can ascertain, she had had the first severe attack of OCD, an illness that she suffers from to this day. Yet in 1961 Roundway Mental Hospital were totally unable to diagnose her illness. Ten years later Charlotte was admitted to the Burden Neurological Institute where Dr. Harry Crow was quick to diagnose and treat the illness as best he could

I can recall many visits to the Burden Neurological Institute in the 1990's. My wife had to attend an out-patients clinic at least four times a year. I suppose that because of the connection with severe mental illnesses. I was often somewhat apprehensive at first on entry. One entered through French windows to reception from a garden. The waiting room was small with about twelve or fifteen upright chairs. Often there were outpatients with severe illnesses, and I often wondered about the safety of Charlotte and myself. Only once can I remember the behaviour of an outpatient, necessitating us to go back into the garden.

The interior was austere and foreboding but nonetheless efficient and clean. I never saw the wards or treatment areas. My wife visited Dr. J. M. Bird, whose office was small and cramped and full, almost to the ceiling with reference books and patient details. Dr. Bird is renowned for his treatment of epilepsy!!

In the early days of Charlotte's treatment her specialist was Dr. Harry Crow, whose main claim to fame was the treatment of mental disorders by surgery. These days specialists prefer treatment byway of drugs. Dr. Crow specialised in selective leucotomy, and has, I believe, written at length on his procedures. It was this operation which was performed upon my wife.

My wife tells me that the initial operation involved the insertion of over fifty wires in the frontal lobes of the brain. Then, about twice a week, an electric current is passed through the wires. The overall effect is that the parts of the brain, which are causing my wife so much distress, are slowly burnt away. Lottie was told, prior to commencement of surgery, that the procedure would never be 100% successful but that there was about a 50/50 chance of progress.

That fifty percent had the effect of saving Lottie's life to say the least. For which my wife will be eternally grateful.

Whilst mentioning the surgical skills of Dr. Crow, I cannot forget Lottie's comments on another aspect of the treatment she received from this remarkable man. As the patient/surgeon relationship grew, Dr. Crow became a father figure to Lottie and never before had she had the advantage of this relationship of a father who she could rely on, to advise her through puberty and all associated growing-up pains that young women undergo.

For instance, he suggested to Lottie that because of her mental conditions, she should not consider parenthood and this advice she heeded, and she has subsequently admitted to me that this action had probably saved her life a second time. So, in many ways the advent of Dr. Crow into Lottie's life was her complete and utter salvation.

No reference to Dr. Crow would b e complete if I did not mention that I have heard that Dr. Crow served with distinction in the Second World War in the Royal Air Force as a navigator in Mosquitos. I believe he retired in the 1980's and died very soon afterwards. This proves to me that he was a truly great man. As I have said I came into contact with the Burden Neurological Institute in the early 1990's and by that time Lottie, who was then an outpatient, was being treated by Dr. Bird. His approach to mental disorder was totally different from that of Dr. Crow. Dr. Bird relied almost entirely on treatment by way of drugs. To give the reader some idea of the regime Lottie has had to endure the regime while she has been with me, her daily drug programme including:

PERCYAZINE 2.5 2 TABLETS 3 TIMES A DAY
FLUOXETINE 20 MG CAPSULES, 1 CAPSULE 3 TIMES A DAY.
PRIADEL 2000 MG 2 TABLETS AT NIGHT
NITRAZEPAM 5 MG 1 TABLET AT NIGHT

This massive dosage has been Lottie's for almost the entire eighteen years that I have known her.

Around the year 2002 the Burden Institute moved from Stapleton to the grounds of Frenchay Hospital with custom built modern premises. Whilst I do not doubt the benefits of this move, the fond memories which people have of the old Burden Neurological

Institute will linger on for some time.

Eventually they will fade completely and I personally feel they should be recorded for posterity, as the Burden Neurological Institute has played such an important part in the advancement of the treatment of some severe mental illnesses.

AN ABANDONED MIND

A few afterthoughts and quotations

I feel that is significant to note that Lottie was one of the last patients to be seen by Dr., Crow immediately prior to his retirement. I think this gesture illustrates the bond which had developed between specialist and patient. I know that Dr. Crow has a special place in Lottie's heart which I know will never diminish.

On a more cheerful note I find that mental health specialists are a rather eccentric breed.

1) Dr.Crow once told Lottie that his wife's maiden name was Sparrow and that when he retired his successor would be Dr. Bird!!
2) Lottie went to see Dr. Smyth on once occasion and Dr. Smyth said to Lottie 'How are you today?' Lottie replied 'Very depressed' - then Dr. Smyth replied 'Oh, so am I'!!

3) Dr. Crow knew of Lottie's love of animals and of dogs in particular. So he told her that he owned two Golden Labrador Puppies and said 'you know, like the ones in the toilet advertisement'!!

Chapter 10 - A New Life for Me

First of all I had my mammogram and this was inconclusive,

Two weeks later I had a call to Swindon General Hospital for a biopsy on my lump with suspected breast cancer.

Three days later I had confirmation of cancer, and removal of this at Salisbury Hospital.

22.05.08 - Operation

23.05.08 - Home with drain for a week and much pain with a district nurse in attendance and also much bleeding, God, how I felt drained! And also sore!

30.05.08 - Back to Salisbury Hospital for drain out and consultation with surgeon, who was very dishy! He put me on anti-eostregon tablets and said that he would arrange to have radiology for a short time.

I cannot say that I would have missed it if I had not had it but I had a wonderful husband and caring sister to take me though these dark days.

I must say that this really was a painful learning curve!!

Poetry

Adolescent poetry

JUST ANOTHER DAY

The sighing breeze, the setting sun
The dewy fields when the night's begun.
The purple clouds, the reddening sky
The stars peep through and the day will die.

But up there in the blue
There's a dream coming true
That will never fade in this earthly shade'

It lingers on, the dream that's come
When the day is gone and the night's begun.

HE'S JUST WONDERFUL (my teacher!!!)

Great his mind, bolt his part
Still I seek the wanted heart
Slender hand and wandering eye,
Ask no question, tell no lie:
Love for sport if loss or gain
Always laugh if sun or rain.
Will it never cease to be
Part of life that dwelt in me!
Will there ever come a time
When that heart will all be mine.
I'm longing for the day that's hoped to be
When he'll be in paradise waiting for me.

AN ABANDONED MIND

ALMIGHTY COMFORT

When darkness spreads its blanket
Gently to the ground.
When birds begin to cease their song
And dew falls to the ground.

The brightness of the day
Sinks 8into darkness of the night
The sun has lost its golden ray
And gone is shining light.

No whisper in the branches
No hustle in the trees.
When human life is sleeping
Tanned by the gentle breeze.

The busy world is silent now;
No more the maddening rush.
All covered by the Mighty Hand
A soothing, warming hush.

Enter into fantasy
Exciting world of dreams
Some frightening, disturbing,
Some bringing hopes and gleams.

No-one can tell what sleep and dream,
What life and Death and silence mean
But when has some life's promised end
We've only turned another bend.

So hope, have faith and know his love.,
For all our lives are planned.

In dark and light take shelter 'neath
His own Almighty hand.

AN ABANDONED MIND

THE YOUNGER GENERATION

No wonder they are drifting, while others cannot
see
Amid the noise and bustle, the ones that are to be.
No wonder they are looking, and yet they cannot
find
The splendour and the glory, the others left behind.

The past is still a burning flame, but they are
turning blind
Toward the darkness a challenge to their mind.
While hoping, waiting, seeking they reach towards
the sky
'Present' still a flame unlit, into the 'past' goes by.

Maybe they'll look, when prime is past, and hairs
are turning grey
Upon a past of peacefulness and to themselves
they'll say
'It's them that made our peace for us,. Moulded
from their world
'But what's in store for those whose lives are yet to
be unfurled.

BURIED ALIVE

Into the winter shadows I must fly
Away from the earth, when the sun must die.
When slender branches bow goodnight
I hide behind them, out of sight.

Blow you cruel wind, your angry breath
Envelopes me with sudden death.
Alone I cry with poignant fear
Alas! No-one but death can hear!

I hail the light, but there below
The graves of sufferers steeped in snow
Are waiting eternity in darkness
And I submit to the earth's caress'

AN ABANDONED MIND

I DIE

Don't forget tomorrow, remember what you said
Don't forget I love you and I will until I'm dead.
The tears I've cried the prayers I've tried
Will prove my heart is true
So make the sun shine through this storm until my sky is blue.

Don't forget tomorrow, rest your hand in mine,
Bestow on me your strength until my soul to yours resigns
Then give me peace and never cease
To love me 'Hear my cry'
"Tomorrow's near, remember dear to kiss me when I die".

US

To those of us, the weak and poor
Deny ourselves the richer score.
We close our hearts, our spirits hide
Falling in our boasting pride.

We shelter where the darkness hides,
Our ,many sins, and all besides.
Though conscience tells when wrong or right
We fail to reach and touch the light.

This weakness is not ours alone
The bravest and the wise have known.
But they've had faith, and they have fought.
Finding happiness they sought.

The moral is for use to see,
That all the world, you and me
If happiness we hope to find.
Faith, love and hope the world can find.'

AN ABANDONED MIND

My poem written for patients at Roundway Hospital when I was twenty one years old:

I pray for you each night
For blessing on your way
And you deserve the happiness
That will be yours one day
Through pain and hurt and sorrow
Despair may often come
But only through life's sufferings
True happiness is won.

The beauty lies around us
Just in the simple things
Be thankful for the blessings
That life for every brings
The word is such a big place
And not all joy and fun
But millions would be glad if they
Like us, could see the sun!!

Sp don't despair in trouble
Just put your faith above
Don't be afraid to stoop and ask
For god's hand and his love
Just let his footsteps guide you
Along the narrow trail.
Until the time that surely comes
When you'll surely live again!

Lightning Source UK Ltd.
Milton Keynes UK
16 February 2010

150162UK00001B/29/P